From Knowledge to Needle

The Path to COVID-19 Immunization

From Knowledge to Needle

The Path to COVID-19 Immunization

Editors: Austin Mardon, Catherine Mardon

Authors: Evangelea Touliopoulos, Ivan Quan, Ivy Quan, and Jenny Gao

Design: Clare Dalton, Ivan Quan

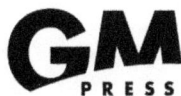

GM PRESS

First Printing: 2020

Typeset and Cover Design by Clare Dalton, Ivan Quan

ISBN: 978-1-77369-167-1

Golden Meteorite Press
103 11919 82 St NW
Edmonton, AB T5B 2W3
www.goldenmeteoritepress.com

Contents

Chapter 1 - The COVID-19 Pandemic

By: Ivan Quan

Death strikes hundreds of thousands and counting. Stock markets crash in the worst economic downturn since the Great Depression. Waves of misinformation spread uncontrollably. Isolation ravages the state of mental health around the world. In other words, COVID-19 takes its first steps, leaving no facet of daily life untouched. As contagious and as widespread as it has become, this disease has forced us to adopt uncertainty as the new norm. For the millions of individuals infected with the disease, respiratory problems, intense pain, and even death is a reality. For the rest of us, cautious of contracting COVID-19, daily routines have shifted to prioritize minimizing the chances of infection.

To prevent disease transmission, large gatherings have largely been abolished. Many employees work from home whenever possible, and non-essential businesses have closed. With the extensive in-person contact occurring in schools, education systems have transitioned to online learning.

Additionally, essential services such as grocery stores have adopted social distancing measures to discourage close contact. Apart from organizations, individuals have also practiced COVID-19 preventative measures. Many have endured self-isolation, only going outside when absolutely necessary. Furthermore, the use of non-medical masks has become routine, and a large emphasis has been placed on keeping physical distance from others. Economically, COVID-19 has caused a global recession comparable to the Great Depression. The instability in supply and demand of goods and services has caused major disruptions to numerous markets. This has devastated the workforce in a large wave of unemployment and reduced labour, with estimates of an overall 14% loss in work hours (International Labour Organization, 2020). Healthcare workers have the opposite problem. Rather than a cut in work hours, the healthcare sector has been greatly overwhelmed by the disease. Many hospitals struggle to provide enough resources to treat the large influx of COVID-19 patients. Hospital bed capacity, personal protective equipment, and other resources have dwindled in supply, especially in developing nations. The increase in healthcare demand has also left many in the industry overworked, with almost 50% experiencing symptoms of depression (Lai et al., 2020). Sadly, the extent of these problems goes far beyond the healthcare industry, as COVID-19 has amplified mental health issues across the population. People with anxiety problems may have found it difficult to cope in these times of uncertainty. Moreover, anxiety may also develop or become heightened due to fear of themselves or loved ones falling victim to the disease. Meanwhile, many practicing self-isolation in an attempt to slow

COVID-19 progression have experienced a decline in social interaction. As a social species, we thrive on connecting with people. Quarantine has taken away this sense of connection, and its effects take toll in the form of high stress levels and depression. Looking at the effects of COVID-19 as a whole, it becomes clear that it is a complex issue with problems manifesting in virtually every aspect of daily life.

A Brief History

To understand how the disease progressed to this point, we must look towards its inception. From the infamous bubonic plague that caused Black Death in the 1300s, to HIV which still affects millions of people today, many of the worst diseases in history have spread to humans from animals (Lloyd-Smith et al., 2009; Sharp & Hahn, 2011). COVID-19 is no exception, originating in bats and spreading to humans in a spillover event (Shereen et al., 2020). A spillover event occurs when a population infected with a pathogen spreads the pathogen to another species. Although the specifics of the COVID-19 spillover event are unknown, the earliest recorded transmissions of the disease occurred in late 2019 at the Huanan Seafood Market in Wuhan, China. COVID-19 was first noticed as a sudden pneumonia outbreak of unknown cause, soon identified to be a symptom of a new strain of coronavirus. As the virus shared many similarities to the SARS-CoV virus that caused the 2003 SARS outbreak, the new virus was aptly named SARS-CoV-2. As the virus quickly spread within China, quarantine restrictions were enforced, suspending transportation within and around Wuhan. Still, COVID-19 managed to spread worldwide, with cases reported in nearby countries like Japan and South Korea, as well as overseas in the United States. On January 30, 2020, with thousands of cases across the globe, the World Health Organization (WHO) declared COVID-19 to be a public health emergency of international concern. This is the WHO's most severe status of alarm, and its justification is clear. As COVID-19 is a novel disease, no vaccines are available to help with immunity. Thus, we must resort to using social distancing measures to restrict transmission of the virus. Staying two meters away from others greatly diminishes the chances of inhaling respiratory droplets. Additionally, many countries around the world have enforced the use of non-medical masks in public spaces. By blocking respiratory droplets from entering the air, they are another effective way to minimize transmission. However, even as countries enforced social distancing measures and travel restrictions, the case count continued to rise exponentially. By March 2020, COVID-19 was categorized as a pandemic as the total number of cases reached 100,000. By April, 1,000,000. By June, 10,000,000 (Dong et al., 2020).

The consistent acceleration in the case count makes it clear—social distancing measures alone are not enough to stop the spread of SARS-CoV-2. Whether it is due to necessary social contact or an ignorance to the virus' dangers, it is apparent that COVID-19 transmission is not slowing. Many essential workers must continue with their jobs, putting them at high risk for infection. Furthermore, many large social gatherings, including weddings, funerals, and in-person conferences, run the risk of becoming a hotspot for mass spread of COVID-19. A single infected person attending a social gathering can transmit the virus to dozens of people in what is known as a superspreader event. Superspreaders propel a significant level of COVID-19 spread, as less than 10% of the infected account for 80% of new cases (Miller et al., 2020). Spread is then further propagated through households, as close contact is almost unavoidable.

The Pathophysiology Behind COVID-19

With the sheer number of infections and deaths caused by COVID-19, a major concern arises. How does the virus infect us and cause disease? SARS-CoV-2 is a coronavirus, appropriately named after the spike proteins present on the surface of the virus that give it an appearance similar to the corona around our sun. When SARS-CoV-2 infects the respiratory system, the disease COVID-19 arises. While infected, coughing, sneezing, and talking expels small droplets of water containing the virus. People nearby may inhale these droplets, giving the virus entry to their respiratory tract through the mouth or the nose. Subsequently, the SARS-CoV-2 virus enters and infects respiratory cells. Many cells in the respiratory system contain the ACE2 surface receptor. The virus' spike protein attaches to the ACE2 receptor, acting as a point of entry into the cell (Yuki et al., 2020). Cell resources are then hijacked to create more viruses. As replication continues, the infected person may remain asymptomatic for up to 14 days. During this time, SARS-CoV-2 is able to evade the immune response and replicate undisturbed. As the quantity of virus grows, it becomes too large to remain undetected from the immune system. As the immune system suddenly becomes overloaded, it rapidly kicks into action, boosting the immune response via inflammation (Rothan & Byrareddy, 2020). When inflammation occurs, blood vessels swell and become more permeable, allowing cells of the immune system to flow into the site of damage. While this can assist with fighting infection, it can also cause an accumulation of fluid (Mcgonagle et al., 2020). The vastly amplified immune response is the cause of many respiratory problems associated with COVID-19, but the symptoms depend on where infection and inflammation happen. Mild manifestations of the disease only involve infection of the upper respiratory tract, which includes components above the windpipe. This can result in a fever, coughing, loss of smell, mild shortness of breath, and a sore throat. More serious manifestations of infection involve the lower respiratory tract (Subbarao & Mahanty, 2020). Pneumonia can arise when the fluid buildup caused by Inflammation occurs in the lungs, restricting air from entering alveoli. The alveoli are tiny air sacs in the lungs that fill with air during inhalation and are crucial for infusing blood with oxygen. In the most severe cases of COVID-19, acute respiratory distress syndrome (ARDS), can occur, involving a rapid widespread lung inflammation that results in respiratory failure. ARDS is the most common cause of death in COVID-19 patients, and its severity means that even survivors will suffer lifelong respiratory issues (F. Yang et al., 2020).

Even though COVID-19's fatality rate is relatively low at a little over 1% when compared to SARS at 10%, the real danger lies in the virus' ability to spread exceptionally well (Petersen et al., 2020). With transmission occurring through respiratory droplets, simply being near an infected individual can lead to inhalation of the virus. Additionally, the virus-containing droplets can land on nearby surfaces. The virus could be transmitted when a person makes contact with the same surface and touches their face. A typical way to reduce rates of transmission would be to quarantine infected individuals. However, evidence shows that COVID-19 is still transmissible during its incubation period (Ye et al., 2020). Lasting up to 14 days, the incubation period occurs between viral infection and the onset of symptoms. This makes it difficult to determine infection status without testing, and contributes to the virus' ease of transmission. Two more factors affecting transmission that go hand in hand, are the viral load of those infected, and the infectious dose required for an infection. Viral load refers to the quantity of viruses present during an infection, while infectious dose refers to the quantity of viruses needed to establish infection. Estimates have put the infectious dose of SARS-CoV-2 to anywhere from 100 to 1000 viral particles (Schaik, 2020). While this is comparable to the infectious dose of SARS at 280 viral particles, it appears that the viral load of SARS-CoV-2 may be up to 1000 times greater than SARS at its peak (Schröder, 2020; Woelfel et al., 2020). A significantly greater quantity of virus is created and released, making transmission much easier.

The COVID-19 Vaccine Story

Though the pandemic situation appears grim, we can find solace in the fact that hundreds of COVID-19 vaccine candidates are in development. As of now, vaccines are the only way to reliably bring the pandemic to an end. In a best case scenario, the vaccine could induce immunity to the disease for a large percentage of the population, slowly eradicating COVID-19 worldwide. There are many aspects to effective vaccination. Certainly, the vaccine must be able to provide protection against the pathogen. In addition, vaccines must be distributed and administered effectively. Not only does this mean that they must be accessible to everyone, it also indicates that those who have access must be willing to use them. The sentiment of vaccine hesitancy, a subject often doused in misinformation, poses a large threat to COVID-19 immunity. As no vaccines are able to provide protection with 100% certainty, a large percentage of the population must be vaccinated to protect communities as a whole.

This emphasis on the importance of vaccines raises

a compelling concern. When will a COVID-19 vaccine be available? A typical vaccine takes 10-15 years to develop, and the mumps vaccine, considered to be the fastest vaccine ever made for a novel disease, took four years of development. Considering this, it seems unlikely that a COVID-19 vaccine would be available anytime soon. However, experts such as Anthony Fauci, the director of the National Institute of Allergy and Infectious Diseases (NIAID) have stated that a vaccine could be ready by early 2021 (Fauci, 2020). A COVID-19 vaccine developed and distributed worldwide with this accelerated schedule could be one of the greatest feats of modern immunology. Not only does this require fast, accurate clinical testing, timely vaccination at such scale also requires an unprecedented level of coordination between vaccine researchers, manufacturers, investors, and distributors. The massive demand for a COVID-19 vaccine has sparked a great race towards immunization, with hundreds of organizations developing hundreds of vaccine candidates. While some vaccines in development employ tried and true traditional methods, others test cutting-edge technology in immunization. Although a vaccine providing immunity to a coronavirus has never been produced, some COVID-19 vaccine candidates have begun to show promising results in clinical trials.

As COVID-19 research flies at breakneck speeds, the vaccine development landscape follows suit, progressing through clinical trials and manufacturing at an unforeseen pace. With the state of worldwide public health under the threat of COVID-19, every small success in vaccine development gives hope towards returning to the normal routines of life. As our best shot at eradicating the global pandemic at hand, let's follow the journey of the COVID-19 vaccine—from knowledge to needle.

Chapter 2 - History of Vaccination

By: Evangelea Touliopoulos

As the pandemic caused by the SARS-CoV-2 virus disrupts society and affects millions of people around the world, one question remains at the forefront of everyone's mind: When will a vaccine be created to put a stop to the COVID-19 crisis? While COVID-19 may have put vaccination in the spotlight for the media and for the general public, humans have been developing and using different forms of vaccination for centuries. This chapter aims to provide a brief overview of the evolution of vaccines and the benefits they provide to society.

The idea of vaccination involves exposure to toxins or viruses in a controlled manner so that the immune system is introduced to the virus without causing the person to suffer the full effects of the disease. This way, should the body be exposed to the pathogen again, the immune system will be capable of quickly responding and fighting the pathogen. Thus, vaccines can provide immunity.

History of Vaccination

While many people may believe that the first experience humans had with vaccination was with the famous smallpox vaccine created by Dr. Edward Jenner, there have been multiple occurrences where the idea behind vaccines was used earlier in history. For example, in 7th century India there have been records in which Indian Buddhists drank snake venom to become immune to the venom's effects (deBary, 1972). While this practice may seem risky and extreme at first glance, it follows a similar principle to modern vaccines; the drinker is voluntarily exposed to the snake venom in a smaller quantity, so if the drinker were to be suddenly bitten by a snake, their body's immune system would be better at dealing with the toxins. This would mean that they will have a significantly less severe reaction compared to if they had no prior exposure to the venom (deBary, 1972). There are also records of the idea behind vaccination being used in China throughout the 18th-century to protect against the smallpox disease (Hume, 1940). Some techniques used included plugging the nose with powdered scabs from those who had been infected with smallpox or to have healthy children wear the undergarments of children who had been exposed to the virus (Leung, 1996). Again, these practices would expose people to the virus to lower their risk of future infection, or in other words, provide potential immunity. While both these methods may seem very removed from the sterile, controlled practices of modern vaccination, they both follow the still used principle of priming the immune system to fight the virus so that the full blown effects of the sickness will not be felt. Although there was more room for error in these dated practices, the benefits of "vaccination" still outweighed the risks.

Another interesting thing about the development of the concept of vaccination is that it was used and recognized by people with no scientific background before it was tested and proven by scientists. For example, many English farmers realized that being exposed to the less deadly cowpox would provide immunity for smallpox (Parish, 1965). One well-recorded case of this was when in the 18th century the English cattle breeder, Benjamin Jetsy, discovered that he was immune to smallpox after contracting cowpox (Parish, 1965). He then decided to intentionally expose his wife and children to cowpox by bringing them to a field where he knew there was a high possibility of contracting the virus (Parish, 1965). This decision provided his children with immunity to smallpox for at least 15 years (Parish, 1965). However, at the time Jetsy was looked down upon for his actions (Parish, 1965). His neighbors were appalled that he would intentionally infect his family with an animal disease (Parish, 1965). Yet, this concept was not completely foreign to the community as it was observed that dairymaids who contracted cowpox would not become sick with smallpox (Parish, 1965). While the reluctance of Jetsy's neighbors to try something that was saving lives may seem silly in hindsight, similar attitudes can still be seen in modern society. There is still a large community of people that are fearful of vaccines and refuse vaccine treatments, even though many members of the anti-vaccination community are well-informed about the possible benefits of vaccines.

The same theory that Jetsy used with his family was later proven to work by the famous English doctor Edward Jenner about 30 years after Jetsy's realization (Pead, 2006). Interestingly,

Jenner came across the idea for vaccines from working as a rural apothecary apprentice and by talking to local dairymaids who knew of how exposure to cowpox could prevent one from contracting smallpox (Pead, 2006). After several experiments, Jenner also realized that cowpox could be passed on from one person to another, meaning that people could be deliberately infected with cowpox (Pead, 2006). This realization provided the groundwork for an early smallpox vaccine using the cowpox virus (Pead, 2006). However, a problem that quickly arose was that immunity from the smallpox vaccine was not lifelong (Parish, 1965). Furthermore, the same strand of cowpox could not be used indefinitely, as it would slowly become too weak to provide immunity (Sherman, 2006). In an attempt to make a stronger vaccine, calves were deliberately infected with the cowpox virus (Sherman, 2006). This allowed the virus to mutate and reproduce in the calf, which meant that there was more vesicle fluid available to be used in vaccines (Sherman, 2006). This allowed for more vaccines to be manufactured and administered to humans (Ballard, 1868). This marked the beginning of the purposeful production of vaccines that are similar to the ones used today. However, these early vaccines were far from perfect. Another problem arose when it was learned that separate bacteria strains, such as syphilis, could contaminate vaccines during the manufacturing process (Copeman, 1899). the bacteria would then be transmitted to people through the vaccine (Copeman, 1899). This led to preservatives and antibiotics being used in vaccines to ensure their safety (Copeman, 1899). For example, Robert Koch's addition of glycerin to the smallpox vaccine helped produce a vaccine that would be safe and consistent (Copeman, 1899).

While Jenner's vaccination technique is a lot more recognizable and comparable to modern vaccines, these early vaccines still lacked formal scientific evidence and testing. Louis Pasteur was the first to conduct successful scientific studies on vaccines that involved controls. This meant that Pasteur tested what would happen to animals that were infected with the virus and compared the results of a vaccinated group vs a non-vaccinated group, called the control group (Pasteur et al., 1881). He conducted this experiment with a potential anthrax vaccine with the goal to prove that vaccination could be conducted systematically. Evidently, Pasteur had success as his animal controls all became ill due to anthrax while the majority of animals from his vaccinated group displayed no symptoms (Pasteur et al., 1881). However, as Pasteur's work expanded to a rabies vaccine, he began working with human subjects. Unsurprisingly, there was an outcry of rage from society regarding the safety of vaccines. When a young boy who had been attacked by a rabid dog was given the vaccine, many people were shocked and furious that Pasteur had deliberately infected a boy with more of the deadly pathogen through vaccination (Pasteur et al., 1881). He faced significant backlash especially when patients died of rabies, even though it was their initial infection that killed them, not the vaccination. Unfortunately, their deaths were attributed to the vaccine even though the patients were vaccinated as a last attempt for rescue (Pasteur et al., 1881). These fatalities were considered to be "medical murder".

Another situation where society protested and fought against the development of vaccines arose shortly after Jenner's development of the smallpox vaccine. The public's fear of being injected with a live virus created a lot of controversy over the safety and the merit of vaccines. This historical fear of vaccines can still be seen today, as there is a growing population who refuse vaccines. In the past, the proven effectiveness of vaccines helped people get over their initial fear of vaccination. This occurred as people came to recognize that experiencing the side effects of vaccines was not nearly as bad as the effects from the real pathogen; as a result vaccines started to become more widely accepted in society. It is for this reason that it is possible that the COVID-19 situation could increase vaccine popularity as the wide scale pandemic caused by the virus proves the necessity of vaccines and demonstrates the harm that occurs when a vaccine is unavailable.

Returning to the development of vaccines, many other vaccines were created after the concept of the smallpox vaccine was discovered. Some important milestones in vaccine development include the vaccines for polio, tetanus, hepatitis A and B, measles, diphtheria, and many more (Centers for Disease Control and Prevention, 2020)! The production of vaccines increased exponentially in the second half of the twentieth century when researchers discovered virus propagation in stationary cell cultures (Chase, 1982). This meant that it was now possible to easily grow pathogens in a controlled manner inside of a scientific lab (Enders et al., 1949). This allowed researchers to safely grow human viruses in vitro to study them and test possible vaccines in a greater capacity (Enders et al., 1949).

Positive Effects of Vaccines

Having all these vaccines revolutionized healthcare and vaccination became integral to improving the quality of human health and increasing the average human lifespan. It is estimated that vaccines have saved over ten million lives between the years 2015 and 2020 (World Health Organization, n.d.)! Having fewer people die from sickness and fewer people being affected by pathogens allowed populations to grow, productivity to increase, and gave people the privilege of living their lives without fearing many of these previously deadly diseases. This enabled the economies of countries to get stronger, for more kids to be able to get educated and for the quality of life in countries with vaccination programs to improve. Evidently, vaccines have really revolutionized the way we live.

Vaccines and Pandemics

While vaccinations are still incredibly useful and effective, they often can be difficult to develop quickly enough to use in pandemic situations for several reasons. A pandemic occurs when a new strand of a virus emerges. Since the specific virus has never been seen in humans before, there will be no immunity and everyone will be highly susceptible to getting infected (Centers for Disease Control and Prevention, 2020). A virus with high pandemic potential will also be able to spread rapidly from person to person, meaning that the number of infected people can increase exponentially. Since vaccines can take a long duration of time to be tested and produced, a pandemic is capable of claiming many lives before an effective vaccine is developed and globally distributed. For example, it took six months to produce a sufficient amount of vaccines for the 2009 H1N1 virus, commonly known as the swine flu. However, there can also be severe consequences when a vaccine is developed too quickly and is not tested thoroughly enough. When paralytic polio became an epidemic in the latter half of the 19th century in Western Europe and the United States, researchers attempted to create a vaccine (Robbins,

2004). Unfortunately, since the vaccines for the paralytic polio were not tested sufficiently, many problems arose including six deaths and many cases of vaccine-induced paralytic polio (Offit, 2005). The public swiftly became scared and outraged by this new vaccine being administered, and unsurprisingly, the production of this first polio vaccine was quickly stopped (Offit, 2005). It took over 15 years before testing restarted, which significantly slowed down the process of developing a polio vaccine (Offit, 2005). Incidents like this are not only tragic and dangerous, but they also slow down scientific progress. Many lives were lost to polio that could have been prevented had a successful vaccine been discovered earlier. Furthermore, these incidents contributed towards a societal fear of vaccines, which can have disastrous consequences if people avoid vaccinating themselves and their families.

The situation involving COVID-19 is a prime example of what can happen when a vaccine for a widespread virus is not available. The first case of COVID-19 can be traced back to November 2020, but a successful vaccine still has not been made as of July 2020. If the absence of a vaccine for just one virus can cause as much havoc as the world experienced since the first SARS-CoV-2 virus case, it is easy to imagine how quality of life would decrease without the existence of vaccines.

To conclude this chapter, it is important to reiterate that vaccination has improved human health immensely. Even though there will always be the small risk of having an adverse reaction involved with vaccination, extensive research and testing has proved that the consequences of not having vaccines are infinitely worse than the potential negative reaction to a vaccine. This is why the concept of vaccination has been used for centuries and why the creations of modern vaccines had the power to revolutionize society by protecting millions of lives from illnesses that were previously severe threats to human health. The devastating effects of the SARS-CoV-2 virus, for which it has taken over eight months to find a vaccine, are a testament to this and should be used as a reminder of the importance and value of vaccination.

Chapter 3 - How do Vaccines Work?

By: Jenny Gao

<u>The Great Vaccinia</u>

It was not until May 8th, 1980 that the variola virus, commonly known as smallpox, was eradicated, as officially announced by the World Health Assembly. This rampaging disease can be traced back to the 3rd century BCE when it originated within the Egyptian Empire. From then, the virus spread globally throughout history until the World Health Organization (WHO) established a plan of action in 1959 for the global vaccination, and in turn the eradication of the virus (Centers for Disease Control and Prevention, 2017). Prior to this initiative, the variola virus killed on average three in every ten persons across the globe due to the virus's complexity in its attacks against the human immune system (World Health Organization, 2017).

As a member of the poxviridae family, the variola virus belongs to a widespread group of brick-oval shaped viruses with double stranded genomes. As with all viruses, their deleterious effects on the human body come from their ability to hijack metabolic machinery in host cells and in injecting their own DNA/ RNA genome for reproduction and survival, and in destroying human host cells in the process.

The variola virus attacks the human immune system and interferes with signal transduction pathways, which is responsible for the binding of internal molecules and invoking a chain of responses in the body (Moore et al., 2006). Between 300-500 million deaths related to the smallpox disease have been recorded over history. So, the complete eradication of smallpox is a propelling feat in history that places emphasis on the necessity of vaccines to support the human immune system. The human immune system (described in more detail later in this chapter) fights off foreign and harmful microscopic particles, importantly known as pathogens. It then commits these pathogenic invasions into their memory to build immunity against future infections (Hopkins, 2020).

In the global initiative plan, the WHO implemented the smallpox vaccinations, accurately named as vaccinia (ACAM2000), to 80 percent of citizens in every country, with a 95 percent success rate in preventing the infection of those who were vaccinated. In just fourteen years, WHO was able to completely eliminate the imminent threat of the smallpox disease that plagued the globe for many centuries. To date, laboratories around the world including France, Germany, Japan, New Zealand and the United States still hold a collective of 31.01 million doses of this vaccine for research (World Health Organization, 2017).

The case of the smallpox eradication highlights the support in which vaccines induce immunity to the human system against deadly pathogens. This chapter explores how vaccines work by delving into the components of the human immune response and its engagement with microbes that may be deleterious to the body.

The Human Immune System

To unravel the intricacy of how a vaccine works, the human immune system must first be understood. The immune system is composed of a network of cells, tissues, and organs that are mapped across various locations throughout the body. These areas include, but are not exclusive to, the nasal, bone, bloodstream, small intestines, abdominal cavity, trachea, spleen and throat. The immune system can be divided into two parts, the innate immune system and the acquired immune system. Inherited from birth, the innate immune system is the first respondent against any microbes that enter the body (Hopkins, 2020). As a primitive system, the innate immune response distinguishes foreign, and potentially harmful, particles from the body's own cells. As a component of the innate system, the first line of defence against microbes include coughing reflexes, enzymes in tears and skin oils, external membrane barriers, mucus and skin/ stomach acid. In addition, there are defense cells from the innate immune system called phagocytes, in particular macrophages, that engulf the invasive microbes in the body (Hopkins, 2020).

In the event that the body's innate immune system is not enough to combat the microbes alone, the acquired immune system provides additional support to help fight off the foreign particles. Phagocytes will bring the digested pathogens in the form of smaller particles, specifically known as antigens, to different cells at the lymph nodes of the immune system that will commit the pathogens to memory (National Institutes of Health,

2020b). From there, the acquired immune system is activated and continues to target the foreign particles. It is under the umbrella of acquired immunity that vaccines work in the body by providing what is artificially acquired immunity.

Acquired Immune System

The acquired (or adaptive) immune system continues to develop upon exposure to the antigens on different microbes that enter the body. An antigen is usually in the form of a type of protein marker that covers a surface region of the invading microbe; the antigen is different for each microbe (U.S. Department & National Institutes of Health, 2008). The antigen itself is the foreign macromolecule that elicits the immune response from the adaptive system. These antigens are similar to identification tags on pathogens in which cells of the adaptive immune cells will recognize. The adaptive immune system is fine tuned in its recognition function, and is able to distinguish between two closely structured antigens of different microbes. There is a specific site of the antigen that the adaptive immune system responds to known as the epitope, which can range from singular sites to multiple areas (Smith-Gill et al., 1984).

While the immune system naturally moves to attack most antigens, the body itself contains the human leukocyte antigens (HLA). These antigens are not attacked by any cells from the immune system because they are not identified as pathogenic particles to the body. In fact, the HLA are located on the surface of most cells in the human body and assist the immune system in distinguishing its cells and tissues apart from foreign molecules (National Institutes of Health, 2020b).

The adaptive immune response is carried out by

two different types of white blood cells including B and T lymphocytes, also simplified as B and T cells. The T cells elicit the cell-mediated immune response and take on both an offensive and defensive tactic in order to detect infected cells. Offensively, the T cells directly attach to the antigen and bind to the epitope, releasing cytotoxic chemicals to kill off the microbe. Defensively, the helper T cells release chemicals to signals for other cells in the immune system to attack the microbe. T lymphocytes also exist as memory T cells that contribute to the adaptive immune response's ability to remember past pathogen encounters and binding to antigens (U.S. Department & National Institutes of Health, 2008). The second type of lymphocytes of the acquired immune system are composed of B cells that elicit the humoral immune response and produce antibodies, or immunoglobulins. Naive and memory B cells will produce specific antibodies to combat the antigens present. These antibodies produced will travel via the bloodstream to infected areas of the body and bind to specific epitopes on the antigen of the microbes (Alberts et al., n.d.).

Anatomy of Antibodies

This subsection takes a brief segue from the immune system pathway to detail the biochemical structure of antibodies and how they bind to a microbe's epitopes, also referred to as the antigenic determinants. In understanding the role that vaccines play in immunization of the human body, it is crucial to break down the foundations of the acquired immune system to the most essential and simplest entities—the antibodies.

An antibody protein is composed of four polypeptide chains fitting into the shape of the letter Y. The top two lines of the letter Y (that open to form a V shape) are the light chains of the protein with amine groups at the end to bind with the antigens. The light chain is further subdivided into the hypervariable region and the framework region. The hypervariable (HV) region, composed of a variety of amino acids, is responsible for the specificity of antibody to antigen binding. The framework region forms beta sheet structures that assist the HV region in effectively binding to the antigen surface.

Some of the antibodies that bind with antigens have the ability to neutralize, in other words, to block the infection in methods such as changing the chemical makeup of the antigen. The antibody could also block the antigen from ever entering into the human host cells and prevent the damage of the microbe's genome. More commonly described, antibodies will mark the foreign intruders to be digested by macrophages or other phagocytes. Antibodies will continue to reproduce for many days following an invasion by pathogens and circulate the body for the many months following.

Reverting back to the pathway of the acquired immune system, there are important B and T cells in the form of memory cells that come into play. Some of the naive lymphocytes from the microbe invasion remaining become T and B memory cells that work to provide the immunity for the body against future attacks from the same pathogens. Note it is because of antibodies that the humoral immune system is a targeted response that allows the processes of vaccines to work against future pathogenic invasions. Both the T and B memory cells are able to store information on the effective stimuli and responses that were carried out by the immune system in destroying the pathogens upon its first exposure. In cases whereby the microbe enters the body again, the T and B memory cells can carry out what is known as the secondary immune response. This immune response is more effective than the first response to the pathogen. During the secondary immune response, B memory cells can elicit quick and strong responses by further differentiating into plasma cells. The functions of the memory cells contribute to the quick production of antibodies that are needed to bind to the antigens (U.S. Department & National Institutes of Health, 2008).

How Vaccines Work with the Human Immune System

Understanding the acquired immune system and its memory functions is crucial to piecing together how vaccines work to provide immunity against certain pathogens. A vaccine is an artificially administered precaution for the human immune system. Essentially, through a simulated-type process, vaccines prepare the body to fend off future invasions of pathogens that will invoke the immune system. Analogous to studying days in advance in order to pass an exam or wearing a seat belt before starting a car for safety in cases of accidents, vaccines work with the immune system to protect the body against future foreign invaders.

In general, a vaccine mimics a potential microbe and tricks the human immune system to respond. Some vaccines may contain weakened or killed versions of a microbe. The vaccine is usually administered by injection into the arm. Since the vaccine form of the microbe has no deleterious impacts, the immune system is easily able to get rid of the simulated pathogen. Upon exposure to the vaccine, the body will produce antibodies and will retain T and B memory cells for immunity against any microbe invasions in the future (U.S. Department & National Institutes of Health, 2008).

Attenuated, Inactivated, Subunit Vaccines and Prime-Boost, Adjuvant Assistance

While the general workings of vaccines have the same foundational effects on the immune system, there are many different types of vaccines in the market. Attenuated vaccines contain weakened, but live, versions of the microbe which enable a strong secondary immune response in future cases of microbe invasions. In contrast, inactivated vaccines are composed of microbes killed by chemicals, heat or radiation. This vaccine type may not be as effective in eliciting the secondary immune response as compared to attenuated vaccines. Subunit vaccines are more fine-tuned and contain only the necessary parts of the microbe (the antigens) to stimulate the body's immune system. Other vaccines include toxoid, nucleic acid, conjugate, and adenovirus vector vaccines (U.S. Department & National Institutes of Health, 2008).

The effectiveness of vaccines can also be improved by using the prime-boost strategy, or by inclusion of an adjuvant. The prime-boost strategy entails the administration of two vaccines to stimulate the immune system's defenses against one microbe species. The first vaccine is used to prime the immune system, usually a DNA vaccine, and the latter vaccine works to boost the effects of the first. In other cases, an adjuvant is added to the vaccine to help increase the vaccine's effects on the immune system. Typically, adjuvants are used in subunit vaccines to keep the antigen stable at the injection sites, or to transport the antigen to locations in the immune system (U.S. Department & National Institutes of Health, 2008).

The Olive Branch of Vaccines

To conclude this chapter on the workings of vaccines to stimulate immunity in the body, it is important to understand how vaccines build from the foundational knowledge of how the acquired immune system achieves memory. Examining the global outbreak of the SARS-CoV-2 virus, working vaccines are essential players in both individual and community health and safety. Aside from the individual immunity provided by vaccines, administering them throughout a community may help in establishing herd immunity. This type of immunity occurs when the majority of a community is vaccinated against a disease. Herd immunity reduces the risks of infection for members in the community that are not able to be vaccinated, such as immunocompromised individuals. In addition to vaccine developments, antiserums and passive immunity are also being researched as a potential solution in the fight against the SARS-CoV-2 virus. Passive immunity is established from passing antibodies between persons by methods such as purified blood known as antiserums (U.S. Department & National Institutes of Health, 2008). In researching antiserum potentials for the SARS-CoV-2 virus, Dr. Davide Robbiani and Dr. Michel Nussenzweig at the Rockefeller University studied blood samples of COVID-19 survivors. In their research, they obtained 149 blood samples, from which 1 percent of samples contained enough antibodies to neutralize the SARS-CoV-2 virus. Preliminary conclusions from similar results obtained on the samples tested state that the antibodies could neutralize the virus by binding to the receptor binding domain on the virus's surface and could prevent the virus from entering the host cell (National Institutes of Health, 2020a).

The ongoing cycle of infection prevention and eradication

by the human immune system highlights the importance of vaccine administration. Vaccine development is therefore an ongoing field of trial and research that is backed by the foundational knowledge of how vaccines work and interact with the immune system.

Chapter 4 - Vaccine Development Process

By: Ivy Quan

Vaccinations are currently the only effective method of controlling epidemics and pandemics in the long-term. Since vaccines are given to healthy people as a preventative measure, they must undergo thorough testing to ensure their safety and efficacy. In this chapter, we will investigate the traditional development of a vaccine from preclinical trials to post-licensure. This meticulous process ensures that all vaccines approved for public use answer three main questions about safety, efficacy, and efficiency. Does the vaccine cause harmful effects in humans, does the vaccine produce the desired immune response, and does the vaccine still work in non-ideal or "real world" conditions? To answer these questions, the vaccine development process can be broken down into five stages. We can think of these stages as the rounds for a rigorous job interview process. Each round will assess the vaccine candidates for safety, efficacy, and effectiveness. These five stages consist of a preclinical phase, phase I, phase II, phase III, and phase IV, or post-marketing surveillance (Singh & Mehta, 2016). The preclinical trials test the preliminary safety of vaccine candidates on groups of cells or animal models to see if the vaccines can be safely administered to humans. Following preclinical trials, the clinical trials consist of phases one through three. These phases involve consecutive increases in sample sizes so that phase I trials consist of tens of volunteers, phase II involves hundreds, and phase III involves thousands. While phase I only recruits healthy adults, phases II and III may involve more vulnerable participants such as children, infants, pregnant women, or people with comorbidities. As such, these trials must follow a strict step-down approach which means that adults are tested first, followed by adolescents, then children, and finally infants. Phase IV is a unique stage because it is ongoing after the vaccine has been approved for marketing. This phase serves as post-marketing surveillance after the distribution of the vaccine to ensure its continual safety by tracking any long-term adverse effects.

Preclinical Trials

Now that we understand the general breakdown of the various stages, it is time to discuss each one in more detail. As mentioned previously, preclinical trials involve animal models, such as mice or monkeys, that are meant to simulate how humans may respond to the vaccine. The primary objective is to assess the safety of the vaccine and to see if it induces an immune response. Sometimes, when ethically permitting, preclinical trials may consist of a challenge trial. Challenge trials test if vaccine candidates actually decrease the risk of infection by intentionally exposing vaccinated subjects to the virus. In June of 2020, researchers at the National Institute of Allergy and Infectious Diseases (NIAID) performed a preclinical challenge trial of a

Middle East respiratory syndrome coronavirus (MERS-CoV) vaccine candidate in chimpanzees. The MERS-CoV vaccine did not show any adverse events, elicited an immune response, and decreased the severity of the infection in vaccinated chimps (Doremalen et al., 2020a). Once researchers are confident that the vaccine candidate is safe for testing on humans, they can progress to phase I of the clinical trials. With this successful challenge trial, the vaccine candidate progressed to phase I of clinical trials in July of 2020 (Folegatti et al., 2020a).

Phase I

The clinical trials mark the commencement of testing vaccine candidates on humans. It starts with phase I trials in which the main goal is to determine the safety and reactogenicity of the candidate. Reactogenicity is simply a word used to describe any short-term side effects of vaccines including fever, and soreness or redness at the site of injection. Secondary goals may include the observation of any immune responses (Singh & Mehta, 2016). Due to these main goals, it is crucial that phase I trials only consist of a small sample of healthy adults with a low risk of infection and a functional immune system. These strict criteria for participants allow researchers to control variables that may contribute to a participant's reaction to the vaccine. Following immunization, participants are closely monitored in a tightly controlled, clinical setting to observe and treat any adverse reactions. All participants also usually undergo blood and urine tests prior to the trial, then throughout and after vaccination to assess any internal changes that may be caused by the vaccine (Singh & Mehta, 2016). Stringent observation is very important for attenuated or inactivated vaccines candidates (which we will touch on in a couple chapters) because they have a risk of mutating to a state that can infect the body. If the healthy adult trial for phase I looks promising, some researchers may perform additional studies on different populations to test how those variables can impact vaccine safety and reactogenicity. However, these variables, such as different age groups, are also accounted for when undergoing phase II trials. To get approved for phase II, vaccine candidates must be safe, must have tolerable reactogenicity, and must generate an appropriate immune response (Singh & Mehta, 2016).

Phase II

Once vaccines demonstrate safety and their ability to stimulate the immune system, the candidates can progress to phase II. Phase II trials are much larger and consist of hundreds of human participants. Due to the large sample sizes, these trials have larger statistical significance. The general purpose of phase II trials is to assess the effect of variables such as ethnicity, age, and sex on safety, reactogenicity, and efficacy. They also commonly provide data to inform the optimal dose, vaccination schedule, and route of administration (Singh & Mehta, 2016).
 Although many vaccines contain the same dosages across different groups, some vaccine dosages may differ for varying reasons. For instance, the shingles vaccine may have higher dosage for adults because the immune system weakens over time. Others, like the tetanus vaccine, have higher dosage for children because each subsequent dose involves a higher risk of arm swelling. Vaccines may also differ by their vaccination schedule. Certain vaccine types may generate a very strong immune response and do not need to be repeated while others need boosters to keep our immune systems alert.
Additionally, researchers may assess different routes of

administration to maximize effectiveness while minimizing the chance of adverse events.

The diphtheria, tetanus, and pertussis vaccine, Tdap in adults and DTaP in children, shows how information about the optimal dose, schedule, and route obtained from phase II trials can impact national vaccine programs. The dosage of the Tdap vaccine in adolescents and adults is approximately two to three times lower than the dosage given to children because older individuals with previous doses of the children vaccine (DTaP) have a higher chance of arm swelling (Centers for Disease Control and Prevention, 2020). Additionally, the dose schedule for vaccines is dependent on many factors. The DTaP vaccine for example, needs a booster dose every ten years because the level of antibodies specific for combatting diphtheria, tetanus, and pertussis will decrease over time (Centers for Disease Control and Prevention, 2020). The route of administration for Tdap and DTaP, similar to many other vaccines, is intramuscular: an injection into the muscle. This is often the most effective method for generating an immune response while limiting unwanted side-effects. Prior to moving onto phase III trials, phase II studies must address how variables such as ethnicity, age, sex, dose, schedule, and route affect vaccine safety and its ability to generate the desired immune response. As such, phase II studies may be conducted in parallel with multiple studies occurring at the same time in different countries.

Phase III and Licensure

The final phase prior to licensure is phase III, which is the largest human trial and recruits thousands of participants with varying levels of health. The large sample size is meant to mimic entire communities of people because the general objective for phase III is to assess how effective the vaccine is at decreasing the number of people who get infected on a population-wide level. To serve this purpose, phase III studies are conducted in communities affected by the infectious disease (Singh & Mehta, 2016). Such locations allow researchers to observe if vaccinated individuals have a lower risk of infection than non-vaccinated individuals: this is called vaccine efficacy. To assess vaccine efficacy, phase III studies are often designed as randomized control trials. These involve participants being randomly selected to receive either the vaccine or a placebo. The placebo is an injection that does not have the active ingredient in vaccines, and will not generate an immune response. If there is no difference in rates of infections between those who were vaccinated and those given the placebo, the vaccine candidate is deemed inefficacious. Randomized control trials can be conducted either single blind, meaning the participants are unaware of which formulation they will receive, or double blind, meaning both participants and researchers are unaware of the formulation during the experiment. Blind trials protect the results from being influenced by human biases during data collection. In randomized control trials, the vaccine candidate can either be tested against a placebo or it can be tested against an existing vaccine to compare their efficacies. Group randomized trials are another way of testing vaccine efficacy. Although not as commonly used as individual randomized control trials, this method allows researchers to assess the indirect effects of vaccines on communities. It can provide information about the percentage of the population that needs to be vaccinated in order to achieve herd immunity (Singh & Mehta, 2016). As discussed previously, herd immunity occurs when those who are not immune are still protected from the infectious disease within their community because enough of the population is vaccinated to prevent disease transmission. Once vaccines demonstrate their safety in large populations and their ability to decrease risk of infection, vaccine manufacturers can submit an application to get their vaccine candidate licensed by a regulatory body such as the FDA. Licensure allows manufacturers to market their vaccines for public use.

Phase IV, Post-marketing Surveillance

Following licensure, vaccines still undergo continual monitoring and re-evaluation. These ongoing studies constitute phase IV trials. The primary goal of phase IV trials is to monitor vaccine safety and effectiveness. While vaccine efficacy measures how vaccines lower risk of infectious disease in ideal and controlled conditions, vaccine effectiveness measures a vaccine's impact on disease risk in non-ideal conditions. As such, phase IV trials are often observational studies that compare the mortality rate or the rate of infection before and after vaccine administration (Hudgens et al., 2004). To continually assess vaccine safety, Health Canada and the Public Health Agency of Canada established the Canadian Adverse Events Following Immunization Surveillance System (CAEFISS). In the United States, the Center for Disease Control and Prevention (CDC) and the United States Food and Drug Administration (FDA) established the Vaccine Adverse Events Reporting System (VAERS). Although they function slightly differently, both CAEFISS and VAERS are examples of federal programs that constantly monitor the safety of marketed vaccines. These programs work to identify previously unknown adverse events, or track the number of reported adverse reactions. Researchers can read the reports released by CAEFISS and VAERS to identify if vaccines need additional investigation.

In 1999, Rotashield, a licensed vaccine for rotavirus, was removed from market due to unforeseen adverse events. Rotashield significantly increased the risk for intussusception in vaccinated infants - a case of bowel obstruction in which the bowel folds in on itself. However, during clinical trials, there was no statistically significant data that suggested the vaccine could cause any severe adverse effects. After cases of intussusception were reported to VAERS, the CDC stopped recommending the vaccine, and its manufacturer withdrew it from the public (Centers for Disease Control and Prevention, 2011). This incident with Rotashield demonstrates the importance of post-marketing surveillance. It is important to note however, that cases such as these are incredibly rare. From January 2013 to December 30, 2018, CAEFISS reported 17 183 adverse events from marketed vaccines, 91% of which were deemed non-serious (Government of Canada, 2019). The rarity of licensed vaccines being deemed unsafe is mostly thanks to the rigorous step-by-step process that vaccine candidates go through to assess their safety and efficacy prior to licensure.

The road through clinical trials is turbulent, and most candidates are unsuccessful. Vaccine candidates undergo meticulous preclinical and clinical testing to ensure that licensed vaccines are safe and elicit an appropriate immune response. Ongoing post-marketing surveillance and phase IV studies then ensure the continual safety and effectiveness of vaccines post-licensure. On average this vaccine development process can last around 10-15 years in total. In an extreme example, the development of the world's first malaria vaccine, RTS,S, took approximately 14 years to progress through the three phases of clinical trials, and took 30 years to get from laboratory development to public availability (RTS,S Clinical Trials Partnership Members, 2015). However, timelines during dire situations such as the COVID-19 pandemic are different. Researchers do not have 10 years to develop vaccines because many people cannot resume regular life without immunity to the infectious disease. In these situations, researchers must find clever solutions to shorten the time frame for vaccine development while maintaining testing quality and participant safety.

Chapter 5 - Vaccine Development During a Pandemic

By: Ivan Quan

Without a global health threat looming over us, the development timeline of a typical vaccine can span 10-15 years. In a pandemic situation, we do not have the luxury to wait such a long time for a vaccine. Less than six months following the first case of SARS-CoV-2 infection, millions have already suffered from COVID-19 (Roser et al., 2020). By the time the typical vaccine development timeline is complete, millions more will be affected and global economies may suffer irreparable damage. During a pandemic, the rapidly growing infection rate pressures the vaccine development process to speed up in various ways. It is crucial to note, that even though the process is accelerated, the goal is still to produce a vaccine with the same safety and efficacy of a typical vaccine.

The Clinical Trial Timeline

In a typical vaccine, each phase of development will happen in consecutive sequence. For example, phase II trials will only be initiated once results from phase I trials are obtained and analyzed. These results must then be reviewed before starting the next phase. However, during the COVID-19 pandemic, many vaccines in development are tested with overlapping steps. Whereas a typical vaccine's clinical trials will strictly progress sequentially, many COVID-19 vaccines start the next clinical phase before completing the previous phase. Moderna's mRNA-1273 vaccine followed this accelerated timeline. Even before phase I preliminary reports were released, the biotechnology company already started dosing phase II and III participants to expedite progression (National Institutes of Health, 2020c).

In addition to running clinical trials in tandem, researchers can strategically combine phases of testing. Usually, combined trials take place in the form of a phase I/II trial, followed by a phase II/III trial. In the combined phase I/II trial, researchers administer varying dosing schedules to hundreds of participants. While the results from these trials can determine the optimal dosage across a range of demographics similar to a typical phase II trial, patients are also monitored for a period of time to test side effects, as in a typical phase I trial. AZD1222, a SARS-CoV-2 vaccine candidate developed by the University of Oxford, conducted this combined phase I/II trial. A variety of dosing schedules and placebos were given to over 1000 participants to assess efficacy, safety, reactogenicity, and to determine the optimal dosage. In the combined phase II/III trial, researchers test the safety and efficacy of the vaccine on a variety of demographics and assess the effectiveness of preventing infection on a wide scale. Together, phase I/II and phase II/III clinical trials cover the same ground as the three phases individually. Although these accelerated systems may not establish the same level of safety for the clinical trial volunteers as the testing of a typical vaccine, the vaccines will still only be licensed after reviewing results from all phases. As the accelerated clinical tests evaluate the same scope as a typical vaccine timeline, this ensures that the final product will be just as safe.

Human Challenge Trials

Normally, challenge trials will be conducted on animals in preclinical trials by intentionally exposing them to the pathogen after vaccination to test vaccine efficacy. However, during the COVID-19 pandemic, many researchers expressed the notion that a human challenge trial could help fast-track vaccine development. In a human challenge trial, volunteers who have received vaccines in a phase II or III trial would be deliberately exposed to SARS-CoV-2, and their condition would be monitored over the course of a few months. A placebo control group, who did not get exposed to the virus but were told that they had, would also be monitored. Results from the placebo would then be compared to the experimental group to determine vaccine efficacy. Whereas traditional phase III trials compare the risk of infection of vaccinated individuals to the unvaccinated over several years, a human challenge trial could cut that time down to several months. Many are pushing for human challenge trials to take place for vaccines against COVID-19, including the organization 1Day Sooner, who is recruiting volunteers to sign up for them. As they are not affiliated with any researchers looking to carry out such a trial, they are simply trying to convince policymakers and the public that it is a viable option with legitimate benefits. Tens of thousands of people signed up for 1Day Sooner, and while no plans exist to carry out this exposure, it proves the willingness of volunteers. Their intent is also to provide a resource for consensual human test subjects in possible future trials (Callaway, 2020). Of course, this poses the ethical concern of weighing the drawback of causing possible harm to participants, with the benefit of accelerating the vaccine development process (Jamrozik & Selgelid, 2020). Although the volunteers would be watched carefully with medical professionals by their side, the possibility of infection still remains if the vaccine is ineffective at preventing the disease. Recognizing the potential advancements that could be made, the World Health Organization (WHO) released a statement outlining the criteria for an acceptable challenge study. Their main reason to consider human challenge trials is because the COVID-19 pandemic poses a great threat to global health, and that gaps in knowledge in regards to the effectiveness of vaccine candidates present a major barrier for public health response. An effective human challenge trial should be able to speed up vaccine development and ensure that the end product works as intended. The WHO also outlines that such a controversial study must be reviewed by a third party expert committee to prevent biases from influencing the conclusion of the study. Only under the conditions that a human challenge study is justified in its potential benefits, is well communicated and coordinated, reduces risk as much as possible, is reviewed by an independent committee, and gets informed consent from volunteers, will it be deemed ethical by the WHO (World Health Organization, 2020b).

Starting Manufacturing Early

In addition to compressing the clinical trial phases together and utilizing human challenge trials, the vaccine production timeline during a pandemic is accelerated by building and preparing factories for vaccine manufacturing during clinical trials. In a typical vaccine without the time restraint posed by a pandemic, organizations would only start looking into manufacturing after the vaccine is approved. Starting the manufacturing process during clinical trials is a huge financial risk because the vast majority of vaccine candidates have issues preventing them from being licensed. This can make many of the premature factory preparations futile. Different types of vaccines require different manufacturing processes, and the infrastructure necessary for production differs depending on the vaccine being produced. This attests to the fact that many of the factories built to produce COVID-19 vaccines will not be able to produce a functional vaccine, and will be inoperative. However, this is the price we must pay for timely vaccine development and distribution. With such preparations, mass-production of vaccines can occur in tandem with clinical trials. Even without a proven vaccine, companies across the globe already have solutions for manufacturing a potential COVID-19 vaccine. Factories in Europe and India committed to producing two billion doses of AstraZeneca's AZD1222 vaccine, and the China National Biotec Group (CNBG) assembled factories developing an unproven inactivated vaccine (AstraZeneca, 2020). The Bill and Melinda Gates Foundation also funded the completion of seven factories for seven possible vaccine candidates, but have stated that they expect that only one or two factories will end up being used to make an approved vaccine (Hamilton, 2020). Even though this will undoubtedly blow billions of dollars, it saves the time of waiting to see which vaccine is functional before production, which could save millions of lives.

Financial Backing

Immense expenditure towards developing a SARS-CoV-2 vaccine is only possible due to a comparably massive amount of funding. The COVID-19 pandemic has resulted in a huge financial push to see a vaccine progress to market. Countries and corporations across the globe are ensuring that organizations developing vaccines have enough funding as well as the financial incentive to do so in the first place. Since many vaccine candidates fail, funding is usually only given to those that have already gone through much of the testing, or seem likely to succeed from preliminary results. Additionally, vaccines designed to be produced for lower-income regions are unlikely to return large profit, as prices must be kept low to support extensive distribution, which discourages financial investment (Snyder et al., 2011). Adequate funding encourages organizations to pursue effective COVID-19 vaccines, and helps cover expensive research and clinical trials. The effects of this funding is clearly demonstrated by the numerous factories committed to vaccine manufacturing even before an approved vaccine. Whereas a typical vaccine manufacturer would never take such a risk, the massive financial backing makes these premature factories possible.

A Look at the Vaccine Candidates

Another angle at which funding has affected vaccine production can be seen in the sheer number of vaccines being developed to combat the pandemic. In response to the global health emergency, hundreds of vaccine candidates have started development. This massive number of candidates is historically unprecedented, and maximises the probability of success. Considering that the vast majority of vaccines do not make it to market, having this many vaccines raises the chance that at least one gets approved. With widespread disease threatening lives around the world, the spotlight is on vaccines as a means to prevent infection, justifying the large financial backing that COVID-19 research and vaccine development has received. A look at the vaccines being developed also reveals that a wide variety of experimental technologies are being considered. From adenovirus vectors, to RNA, to DNA vaccines, none of these platforms have ever been approved for use as a human vaccine, yet over 50 candidates are in the works. These revolutionary technologies could prove useful to immunology, as no traditional vaccine has ever been successfully produced to provide immunity to any form of coronavirus (Padron-Regalado, 2020). Because of the uncompromising time frame set by the COVID-19 pandemic, it is worth pursuing a wide variety of vaccines, including next-generation approaches. Being on the cutting edge, novel methods can offer benefits such as massively increased production speed and lowered costs, but may prove challenging to develop (Le et al., 2020). Regardless of a successful outcome, the technology used will undoubtedly pave the way for the future of vaccination.

What if the Pandemic Ends?

A curiosity that could arise is the question of what would happen to vaccines in development, if the pandemic situation is controlled before a vaccine is approved. We can look at past outbreaks to reflect on possibilities. Historically, many vaccines in development have experienced sharp cuts in funding after the largest waves of infection ended. During the 2015–2016 Zika virus epidemic, dozens of vaccines were in development, including an inactivated vaccine developed by French company Sanofi and the Walter Army Institute of Research. As Zika was declared as a "public health emergency of international concern" by the WHO in early 2016, organizations rushed to find solutions to the outbreak (World Health Organization, 2016). This inactivated vaccine, funded by the U.S. Biomedical Advanced Research and Development Authority (BARDA), had shown great promise in a phase I clinical study (Modjarrad et al., 2018). During its development, the spread of the Zika virus had slowed considerably. In turn, BARDA reacted in 2017 by pulling funding from the venture, and Sanofi consequently halted development of the vaccine. Though development was stopped in a way that it could be restarted if another Zika outbreak arose, it would still take plenty of time before a vaccine could be brought to market (Sanofi, 2017). A similar situation happened with the 2003 SARS outbreak.

While attempts at creating a vaccine had been made even as recently as 2016, there was little interest in financially contributing to their success. A team of researchers at the Texas Children's Hospital developed a SARS vaccine candidate ready for clinical testing, but with the previous SARS outbreak being years past, no one was willing to support it. As such, they were forced to abandon their project. If the COVID-19 pandemic ends before a successful vaccine is made, it is possible that the vaccines in development could suffer the same fate. Without interest, financial support is unlikely, rendering the hope of further development and clinical trials inconceivable. However, it should be in the public interest that these vaccines still continue with investigation. This way, in the event of a future outbreak of the disease, or one that is similar, we will be more ready to react with immunization. A successful SARS vaccine could have helped greatly with the progress of a COVID-19 vaccine due to their similarities. Even so, in their unfinished states, previous efforts on a SARS vaccine has given valuable information to assist researchers in the construction of a vaccine against COVID-19.

Chapter 6 - Comparing Three Coronaviruses

By: Evangelea Touliopoulos

  While the recent pandemic caused by the SARS-CoV-2 virus was unprecedented in multiple ways, the SARS-CoV-2 virus has not been the first coronavirus to infect humans. While the idea that there are other strains of coronaviruses may seem disheartening, these other coronaviruses provide researchers, healthcare professionals, and policymakers something with which to compare the SARS-CoV-2 virus. By comparing similarities and differences, researchers can have a better understanding of possible treatments and vaccines for the virus, as well as what might not work. The two coronaviruses that have had the biggest impact on humans besides SARS-CoV-2 have been SARS-CoV and MERS-CoV (Rabaan et al., n.d.). In the rest of this chapter, we will uncover similarities and differences between the three viruses and investigate how these comparisons help with the development of a vaccine.

General Overview of the Three Viruses

A coronavirus is an enveloped, positive single-stranded RNA virus (G. Li et al., 2020). This means that it is a virus with its genetic material wrapped in a protein 'envelope' and that its genetic material is one strand of RNA that is already ready to be replicate (G. Li et al., 2020). Furthermore, coronaviruses are characterized by their spike proteins on the surface of the virus. These spikes are proteins that resemble a crown, hence giving them the name 'coronavirus' (G. Li et al., 2020).

Human Coronavirus Structure

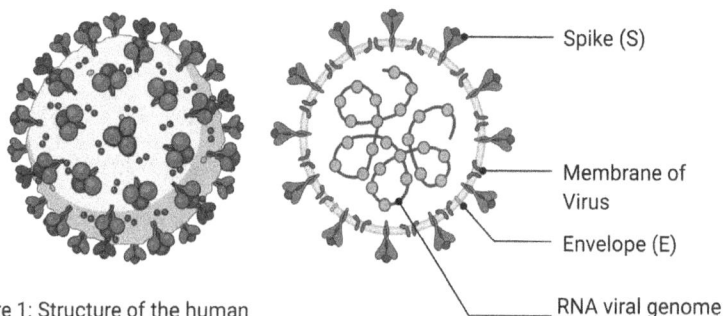

Spike (S)

Membrane of Virus

Envelope (E)

RNA viral genome

Figure 1: Structure of the human coronavirus showing the spike proteins on the surface of the virus and the RNA viral genome. Created with BioRender.com

The first of these three coronaviruses to infect humans was the SARS-CoV virus which first emerged in November of 2002 in the Guangdong province of China (Rabaan et al., n.d.). This virus is thought to have originated from bats (Rabaan et al., n.d.). From the bats, the SARS-CoV virus infected civets, a small mammal native to tropical Asia and Africa (Rabaan et al., n.d.). When the civets were sold in a live animal market in Guangdong, the virus was transmitted to humans, beginning its spread from person to person (Rabaan et al., n.d.). The SARS-CoV virus had a mortality rate of 9% (Rabaan et al., n.d.). This means if 100 people were to be infected with the virus, nine of them would die. However, the mortality rate would be higher among elderly populations and those who have compromised immune systems because they are less able to fight the virus and remove it from their systems once they have been infected (Rabaan et al., n.d.). The SARS-CoV virus causes a respiratory infection with similar symptoms to pneumonia such as difficulty breathing and inflammation in the lungs. The virus will use the ACE2 receptor to be able to enter cells, such as the lungs' epithelial cells (Rabaan et al., n.d.). Furthermore, since it affects the lungs' epithelial cells as well as immune cells, such as macrophages and dendritic cells, elevated levels of cytokines are produced (Rabaan et al., n.d.). Cytokines are small protein molecules that are released from cells to communicate with one another (J. Zhang & An, 2007). In the case of a viral infection, the cells will release cytokines that can elicit various effects on many different cells throughout the body (J. Zhang & An, 2007). Having elevated levels of cytokines means that the patients will experience systemic (full body) effects from the virus (Rabaan et al., n.d.).

The Middle East Respiratory Syndrome Coronavirus (MERS-CoV), emerged from Saudi Arabia in April 2012 and is also thought to have originated from bats (Rabaan et al., n.d.). However, instead of the bats infecting civets in a similar fashion to the SARS-CoV, the bats transmitted the virus to camels, which are common animals in the Middle East (Rabaan et al., n.d.). People were then infected if they ate contaminated camel meat or milk, or if they touched camels that were infected (Rabaan et al., n.d.). There was also limited human to human transmission, but only through close contact. Out of the three viruses, MERS-CoV had the highest mortality rate (Rabaan et al., n.d.). When it first originated it had a mortality rate of about 50%, but as it continued to spread and evolve, the mortality rate dropped to about 34%, which is still significantly higher than the mortality rate for SARS-CoV (Rabaan et al., n.d.). Since MERS-CoV is also a respiratory infection, difficulty breathing, a cough, and a sore throat are some of the most common symptoms (Rabaan et al., n.d.). However, while MERS-CoV affects many of the same cells as SARS-CoV, it binds with a different receptor: the DPP4 receptor (N. Wang et al., 2013).

Finally, the infamous SARS-CoV-2 virus emerged in Wuhan, a city in the Hubei province of China. The first cases were seen in late November 2019, but the virus was identified as something atypical and potential dangerous in December of 2019 (Rabaan et al., n.d.). Similar to SARS-CoV, SARS-CoV-2 originated from bats and is thought to have been transmitted to humans at a live animal market in the city of Wuhan (Rabaan et al., n.d.). While the intermediate vector between bats and humans is still not proven, many hypothesize it to be pangolins, which are mammals that are eaten in China and were sold at the live animal market in Wuhan (Rabaan et al., n.d.). What many people do not expect is that SARS-CoV-2 has the lowest mortality rate when compared to SARS-CoV and MERS-CoV (Rabaan et al., n.d.). While there are a variety of estimates on the mortality rate of COVID-19, the disease caused by the SARS-CoV-2 virus, the most common estimates claim that it is between 0.9% and 2% (La Vignera et al., 2020). The SARS-CoV-2 virus also primarily infects the respiratory tract and has similar symptoms to the SARS-CoV virus. It even uses the same receptor as the SARS-

CoV virus, ACE2, to enter human cells (Rabaan et al., n.d.).

One thing that is interesting to note about the three viruses is that the number of fatalities of each virus are not directly related to the virus's mortality rate. Even though SARS-CoV-2 has the lowest fatality rate of the three viruses, it has many more fatalities than SARS-CoV and MERS-CoV, which both have under 1000 fatalities each (Center for Disease Control and Prevention, 2005). This is because the SARS-CoV-2 virus is much more transmissible (Rabaan et al., n.d.). The virus' contagious nature can be attributed to its longer incubation period, which is the time when a person is infected with the virus but not presenting any symptoms (Lauer et al., 2020). Furthermore, the symptoms are less severe. This means infected people are less likely to realize they are infected and more likely to continue their daily routine while infected with the virus. As a result, the number of people who became infected by the SARS-CoV-2 virus and who developed COVID-19 is exponentially higher than the people who contracted either SARS-CoV or MERS-CoV (Rabaan et al., n.d.). Because of this, COVID-19 will have a higher death count even with its lower mortality rate.

Structural Similarities and Differences Between SARS-CoV-2, SARS-CoV, and MERS-CoV

Now that we have an understanding of the basics of the three coronaviruses that have had a significant impact on humans in the last two decades, we need to understand the structural similarities and differences between the viruses, as this will be helpful when developing possible vaccine candidates.

SARS-CoV-2 and SARS-CoV have a very similar structure with genetic similarity of 79%, which is greater than the genetic similarity of SARS-CoV-2 and MERS-CoV, which is only

50% (Rabaan et al., n.d.). However, one significant difference is that the S protein of SARS-CoV-2 is longer than both the S proteins of SARS-CoV and MERS-CoV (Rabaan et al., n.d.). The S proteins are the spikes on the surface of a coronavirus that give it its crown-like appearance. They are also responsible for binding to the ACE2 receptor and for helping the virus gain entry to human cells (Rabaan et al., n.d.).

Coronavirus Structure and S Protein Visualization

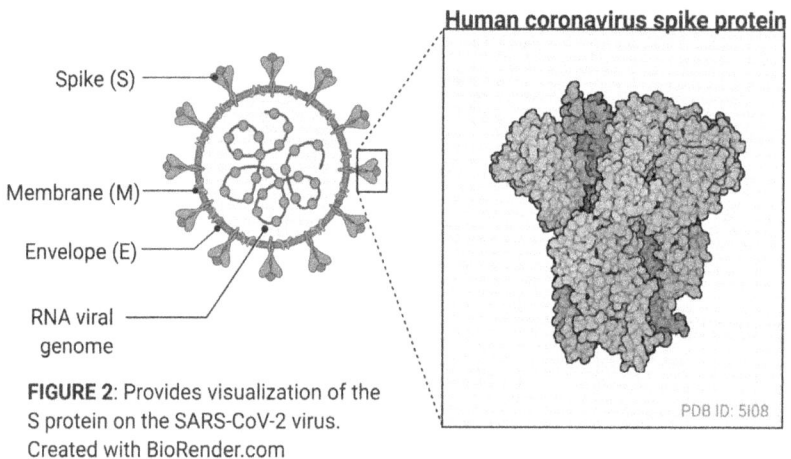

FIGURE 2: Provides visualization of the S protein on the SARS-CoV-2 virus. Created with BioRender.com

The part of the S protein that actually attaches to the receptor (ACE2 for both SARS-CoV-2 and SARS-CoV) is appropriately called the receptor-binding domain (RBD) (Q. Wang et al., 2020). The SARS-CoV-2-RBD exhibits 73.9% structural homology to SARS-CoV-RBD (Q. Wang et al., 2020). This high degree of homology is reflected in their many similar features. Of the 14 amino acids that the SARS-CoV-2-RBD uses to bind to the ACE2 receptor, 8 are the same in the SARS-CoV-RBD (Q. Wang et al., 2020). However, that means there are 6 different amino acids between the RBDs of the two viruses.

These non-conserved amino acids can account for some of the differences in pathogenicity and transmissibility between the two. For instance, one of the amino acids in the SARS-CoV-RBD is leucine, but in SARS-CoV-2, leucine is replaced with the amino acid phenylalanine (F. Li, 2014). The phenylalanine will form stronger interactions with the amino acid tyrosine in the ACE2 receptor (F. Li, 2014). This will occur because both phenylalanine and tyrosine have a benzene group (F. Li, 2014). These two benzene groups will be strongly attracted to each other, which means there will be a stronger bond between the S protein and the receptor (F. Li, 2014). These changes in the amino acids in the RBDs mean that SARS-CoV-2 and SARS-CoV will bind to the ACE2 receptor with different levels of stability. Since the interactions are stronger between the amino acids on the SARS-CoV-2 virus and the ACE2 receptor, it is thought to bind to the receptor with four times more strength than SARS-CoV (F. Li, 2014). Having this more stable interaction means that it will be easier for SARS-CoV-2 to enter the cell compared to SARS-CoV.

Interaction between S protein of SARS-CoV-2 virus and ACE2 receptor

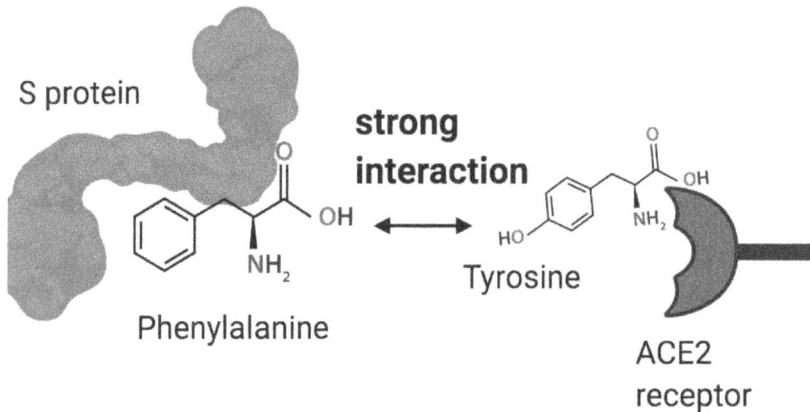

Figure 3: The amino acid phenylalanine on the S protien of the virus and tyrosine on the ACE2 receptor have a strong interaction allowing the virus to bind to the receptor. Created with BioRender.com

After the virus binds to its receptor, the S protein needs to be cut into its S1 and S2 subunits (Rabaan et al., n.d.). This cleavage is essential for the virus to be able to fuse with the cell to release its genome, and it is therefore integral for its reproduction (Rabaan et al., n.d.). Both SARS-CoV and SARS-CoV-2 use a furin enzyme to cleave their S proteins (Rabaan et al., n.d.). An enzyme is a small protein molecule that will significantly lower the amount of energy needed for a reaction to occur, which allows the reaction to occur faster. MERS-CoV also has a S1/S2 cleavage site, but furin mediated cleavage is much less favourable for this virus (Rabaan et al., n.d.). This is another example of how SARS-CoV and SARS-CoV-2 are much more similar to each other than to MERS-CoV.

By understanding these structural comparisons, we can start to look for ways that we can target and use the structure of the SARS-CoV-2 virus to allow the body to develop immunity to the virus. This knowledge is therefore integral for vaccine production.

Possible Vaccination Options for COVID-19

One potential target for a COVID-19 vaccine could be furin inhibitors (Rabaan et al., n.d.). This would be a logical target because furin inhibitors could prevent the cleavage of the S1 subunit from the S2 subunit (Rabaan et al., n.d.). Without this cleavage, the virus would not be able to enter the cell and would not be able to reproduce.

Another possible way to mitigate the effects of SARS-CoV-2 virus would be to develop a vaccine that targets the RBD. As discussed earlier, the RBD of the SARS-CoV-2 virus plays an essential role in the virus's ability to enter cells and reproduce. If the body develops antibodies that target the RBD of SARS-CoV-2, then the immune system would be able to quickly eradicate the pathogen if it ever comes into contact with it again. It is for this reason that subunit vaccines have a lot of potential. Subunit vaccines are composed of a specific piece of a pathogen that will be used to activate an immune response (Clem, 2011). This will then give the body acquired immunity against the pathogen from which the vaccine is derived. Understanding the structural composition of the SARS-CoV-2 virus is incredibly important in the search for a subunit vaccine, as it is imperative for researchers to know exactly what protein they are trying to produce. Subunit vaccines for COVID-19 hold a lot of promise and many are already in advanced stages of clinical trials as we will discuss in a couple chapters. Another type of vaccine that can stimulate production of the antibodies found on the S protein is a RNA vaccine, which is a vaccine that uses modified and synthetically created viral RNA (Clem, 2011). The RNA sequence will then code for proteins that are often identical to a fragment of the pathogen of interest (Clem, 2011). An example of an RNA vaccine that shows a lot of promise is Moderna's mRNA-1273 vaccine. In Moderna's case, the synthetic RNA resembles a sequence relating to the spike protein of the COVID-19 virus (Moderna, Inc., n.d.). Once our immune systems have been exposed to the spike protein, our immune cells will store a memory of the virus and will then be ready to quickly eradicate it if the same protein ever poses a threat again. The Moderna vaccine is just one example of the many vaccines that target the spike protein and are currently being tested for their ability to provide immunity against the SARS-CoV-2 virus.

Significance of Comparing the Three Different Coronaviruses

Evidently, by examining the similarities between the different coronaviruses, we are able to have a better understanding of the SARS-CoV-2 virus. This knowledge can also provide us with potential vaccine targets. Considering the positive effects that finding a vaccine for COVID-19 would have, it is important that we utilize all the resources available. Comparing SARS-CoV-2 to previous coronaviruses, such as SARS-CoV and MERS-CoV, helps to provide an understanding of our adversary that is as complete as possible.

Chapter 7 - Live-Attenuated and Inactivated Vaccines

By: Jenny Gao

On January 11th, 2020 the World Health Organization released the genetic sequence of the SARS-CoV-2 virus to the public. Seven months later, over 180 vaccines were being developed globally. The immense quantity of coronavirus vaccines candidates is advantageous because of the diverse vaccine technology platforms being developed (Lee, 2020). To choose the most suitable vaccine platform, researchers look at how each vaccine type stimulates the immune system and the safety of the vaccine for those receiving it (World Health Organization, 2017). In addition, vaccine developers must consider adjuvants to help enhance the immunogenicity of less effective vaccine types which may be used for patients with compromised immune systems

In this chapter we will focus on two of the most traditional types of vaccines available for development, live-attenuated vaccines and inactivated (killed) vaccines. Both forms are conventional vaccine platforms used to eradicate and prevent various types of diseases. We will explore the advantages and risks of both types of vaccines by investigating their contribution to past disease prevention efforts. We will also highlight the research that has been conducted on live-attenuated and inactivated vaccines against the COVID-19 virus.

Live-attenuated Vaccines

Live-attenuated vaccines use live, weakened forms of pathogens that cause the disease. This vaccine technology platform mimics the natural infectious pathogen with great accuracy. Due to its resemblance to the actual pathogen, live-attenuated vaccines are advantageous because they can induce a very strong immune response. Since it elicits such a strong response, the body can develop a long-lasting immunity against the pathogen and therefore a person may require only a single dose of the vaccine. This will be an important advantage for the mass distribution of the COVID-19 vaccine if it were a live-attenuated platform. Live-attenuated vaccines have been used to protect the human immune system against pathogens such as measles, rotavirus, chickenpox, yellow fever, wild poliovirus, and smallpox (World Health Organization, 2017).

In chapter three, we emphasized the important role of the vaccinia virus used in the smallpox vaccine in the eradication of the variola virus. In its earliest forms, the smallpox vaccine was administered in a process known as variolation. This process extracted the pustular (infected) material from a person with smallpox and then inoculated it into another individual for immunity against the disease. Inoculation refers to the introduction of a pathogenic substance into the body in order to induce immunity; in this sense, vaccination is a form of inoculation. In the 1600s, Dr. Edward Jenner delivered this form of live-attenuated vaccine by breaking the outer skin layer on the upper arm of a patient with a lancet and then rubbing the smallpox material into the lesion (Belongia, 2003). In the 1960s, the live smallpox vaccine was administered via a bifurcated needle, a two-pronged steel rod. There were three generations of the vaccine put forth by the WHO. The first and second generations of the vaccine used inoculated strains of the variola virus derived from the skins and lymph nodes of animals. These generations were used during the most intensive eradication period of the smallpox disease (World Health Organization, 2017).

While live-attenuated vaccines are advantageous in inducing a strong immunity, there are inherent health risks that come with it. The safety concerns of live-attenuated vaccines arise from their ability to revert to their pathogenic forms because the vaccine still uses living forms of the disease. Therefore, live-attenuated vaccines cannot be used by people with compromised immune systems. This includes people who have HIV/AIDS, leukemia, lymphoma, inherited immunodeficiency, organ transplants, cancer, or those who are pregnant. Additionally, since the vaccines are inoculated in the tissue cultures of animals, there is a risk that the animal tissue contains other potentially harmful viruses. Live-attenuated risks from the smallpox vaccine can be seen through the rare, but harmful effects from the administration of the smallpox virus strains. Abnormal adverse effects from the smallpox vaccine ranging from minor to severe lesions, fever, muscle aches, inflamed lymph nodes, fatigue, headaches, and nausea were recorded in some vaccinated individuals. Rare cases of progressive smallpox in those vaccinated were also recorded, which means that the virus in the vaccine replicated uncontrollably at the site of injection and led to the premature death of host cells. Therefore, researchers and clinicians must consider these advantages and disadvantages when developing and administering live-attenuated vaccines. While additional research must be conducted for COVID-19 vaccine candidates, the transmission of a weakened, but still live, version of the SARS-CoV-2 strain in a vaccine may not be appropriate to administer for patients who have immediate family members with compromised immune systems, and therefore another type of vaccine may need to be considered (Belongia, 2003).

Bacillus Calmette-Guérin (BCG) Vaccine

As we briefly touched on the risks of administering an attenuated version of the SARS-CoV-2 virus strain as a vaccine, there arises another microorganism, a bacterium strain, that may be used to reduce the severity of a coronavirus infection. While the Mycobacterium is not a coronavirus strain, it is a bacterial pathogen used in the Bacillus Calmette-Guérin (BCG) vaccine against tuberculosis. To emphasize, the BCG vaccine is not a live attenuated version of the SARS-CoV-2 virus strain used in a vaccine, but research has been conducted on the BCG as a method of fighting against COVID-19. In 1921, the BCG vaccine was developed at the Institut Pasteur in Paris to fight against tuberculosis, an airborne infectious disease that attacks the lungs. While not yet recommended by the WHO, the BCG vaccine has been loosely correlated to reducing infections of the respiratory tract, which may assist in the fight against the COVID-19 pandemic (O'neill et al., 2020).

Beginning in the 1920s, randomized studies on 130 infants concluded that this live-attenuated vaccine reduced infant mortality caused by blood infection pathogens, which was not specifically from the Mycobacterium bacteria that causes tuberculosis. Research conducted in Guinea-Bissau, West Africa also links a reduction in some respiratory and blood infections in youth vaccinated with BCG. Further research in Indonesian elders and clinical trials in Japan also suggests a reduction in respiratory tract infections of those with BCG vaccinations. Randomized studies on the immunity provided by the BCG vaccine have found that the attenuated Mycobacterium strain induces protection in the immune system against various respiratory diseases including syncytial virus (RSV), influenza A virus and herpes simplex virus type 2 (O'neill et al., 2020). The question that best lends itself to finding a coronavirus vaccine is: Why might a BCG vaccine reduce viral infection when it was originally targeted towards a bacterial disease?

While much of the vaccine research on the novel coronavirus emphasizes studies on antibody production against viral pathogens, the BCG vaccine is advantageous because it boosts the performance of our innate immune system instead. The administration of the BCG vaccine triggers the production of proinflammatory and anti-inflammatory cytokines, along with cytokine inhibitors that enhance the innate immune system's response. Cytokines are signaling protein molecules in the immune system that are responsible for regulating immunity and inflammatory responses. While temporary, the BCG vaccine is effective in enhancing the response of phagocytes in the innate immune system. The BCG vaccine induces a trained immune response in the body through epigenetically upregulating the response of the innate system's cells and molecular structures involved (O'neill et al., 2020).

Epigenetic Reprogramming

Epigenetic reprogramming can either increase or decrease the transcription of genes and can in turn, enhance the innate immune responses. Genes are short sections of our DNA containing the instructions to code for the proteins needed in our cells. The cells in our body are flexible and highly efficient in changing their physiological and molecular identity through the genes that are expressed. It is important to note that in epigenetic reprogramming, our DNA sequence and genome is never changed. Instead it is how easily our genome can be transcribed by host cell machinery that changes. We can think of modifying the epigenome through the coiling of the DNA. Following the administration of the BCG vaccine, the histone proteins that regulate chromosome (DNA) condensation (coiling) and relaxation (uncoiling) are chemically modified. From the physical alteration of the DNA packing, some genes are more easily transcribed, while others are hidden and turned off. In response to BCG, DNA uncoils, exposing pro-inflammatory cytokine genes. As a result, BCG amplifies the amount of pro-inflammatory cytokine protein released. In this epigenetic reprogramming, genes that are necessary for phagocyte responses are exposed for transcription, therefore enhancing the innate immune response (Krishnakumar, 2013).

Cytokines in the Innate Immune Response

Epigenetic reprogramming induced by the BCG vaccine results in an enhancement in the innate immune system's response to respiratory infections and an increase in macrophage response.

Studies with the BCG vaccine have demonstrated an increased amount of proinflammatory cytokines produced in response to the mycobacterium in the body. The proinflammatory cytokines cause inflammation in the infected area, which triggers a chain reaction where anti-inflammatory cytokines enter the scene along with cytokine inhibitors. The cytokine inhibitors will block the actions of both the proinflammatory cytokine and the anti-inflammatory cytokines that were triggered to respond. Through this action in the inflammatory responses, the innate system will be enhanced (Srinivasan, 2017).

As of July 2020, the BCG live-attenuated vaccine is in Phase II/III of clinical trials for its testing as a coronavirus vaccine candidate. Researchers have found that Europe was an epicenter for the coronavirus pandemic, while other low and disadvantaged countries reported lower cases of the coronavirus in civilians. They hypothesized since a lot of the developing countries still mandate the BCG vaccine, there may be a correlation worthy of further investigation (Gursel, 2020). However, it is necessary to mention that as of August 2020, the WHO has not yet recommended the BCG as a suitable vaccine to be used against the COVID-19 virus.

Inactivated (killed) Vaccines

While there is no denying the efficiency that live-attenuated vaccines provide in strengthening the immune system response with long term protection against diseases, it is also hard to overlook the potential harmful effects the vaccine can elicit. Take for instance, the rare, but deleterious effects from the global administration of the Sabin-strain oral polio vaccine type 2 (OPV2) used in the eradication of wild type 2 poliovirus. The

Sabin strain polio virus used was unstable at times and could revert to its pathogenic phenotype, causing permanent damage in the nervous system. After thorough investigation on OPV2, the World Health Organization made the decision in April 2016 to discontinue the use of the live-attenuated vaccine and switch to the inactivated Salk poliovirus vaccine instead (Mccarthy, 2017).

With the urgency to develop a coronavirus vaccine, researchers have to consider using other vaccine technology platforms besides live-attenuated vaccines in order to reduce health risks. This is especially important when considering the accelerated and condensed clinical testing time available during the pandemic. Therefore, an inactivated COVID-18 vaccine candidate may offer a safer pathway to research.

Inactivated vaccines use killed versions of the pathogen that cause the disease. Since this form of vaccine is dead, it can be administered to people who are immunocompromised, giving it an advantage over live-attenuated vaccines. On the other hand, the killed microbe does not mimic its pathogenic version as accurately, and therefore, the induced immune response elicited is weaker than that of a live-attenuated vaccine. Patients getting the inactivated vaccine may have to receive several booster doses throughout the year to remain protected against the pathogen. Inactivated vaccines have been used to protect against and prevent diseases including hepatitis A, rabies, poliovirus, and the seasonal flu ("How Vaccines Work," 2019).

Influenza Vaccine – The Seasonal Flu

Commonly referred to as the flu shot, the influenza vaccine is an inactivated vaccine. This inactivated vaccine is known as a quadrivalent vaccine because it contains four different strains of influenza viruses to help fend off the seasonal flu. These four viruses include influenza A (H1N1) virus, influenza A (H3N2) virus, and two different influenza B viruses. In some cases, a trivalent influenza vaccine is administered with only one type of influenza B virus included. In contrast to the strict safety guidelines of live-attenuated vaccines, the inactivated influenza vaccine is highly recommended for higher risk individuals such as: those that are pregnant, youth, asthmatics, elders, and diabetics. However, individuals with egg allergies should be advised that the viral strains are grown within the embryonic fluids within chicken eggs (Centers for Disease Control and Prevention, 2019).

CoronaVac – Inactivated COVID-19 Vaccine Candidate

Immediately following the release of the SARS-CoV-2 genetic sequence, Sinovac Biotech based in Beijing, China began its research on a vaccine containing a chemically killed form of the SARS-CoV-2 virus. The private biotechnology company harvested SARS-CoV-2 strains from the kidney cell linings of African green monkeys and developed the inactivated CoronaVac vaccine. In preclinical challenge trials, they tested the vaccine on rhesus macaque monkeys. While all monkeys survived the infection, those given higher doses of CoronaVac had a better immune response and a faster recovery compared to monkeys given lower doses (H. Yang, 2020). However, scientists globally were quick to point out that the novel coronavirus administered in the monkeys may not be representative of how the human immune systems would respond to the vaccine. On the other hand, continued testing of CoronaVac during preclinical trials has been promising. The antibodies taken from the monkeys, rats, and mice that participated in the challenge trials successfully neutralized the coronavirus strains upon exposure. After a phase I/II clinical trial was conducted on over 1000 human volunteers, Sinovac Biotech moved onto phase III of clinical trials (Cohen, 2020). On July 3rd, 2020, the biotechnology company announced its collaboration with Butantan, an immunobiological production company in Brazil, after gaining approval from the Brazilian National Regulatory Agency for phase III of clinical trials. During phase III, CoronaVac will be distributed to twelve clinics in Brazil as approved by an agency vetted through the World Health Organization (H. Yang, 2020).

With the available selection of different platforms for vaccine candidates, researchers and scientists can assess different strategies to develop a working novel COVID-19 vaccine. Live-attenuated and inactivated coronavirus vaccine candidates exemplify the different vaccination types and technologies being considered. The broad preventative effects that the live-attenuated Bacillus Calmette-Guérin vaccine may offer against the SARS-CoV-2 highlights how enhancing the innate immune system may help against COVID-19. Moreover, the inactivated vaccine CoronaVac developed by Sinovac is a modern example of a traditional vaccine technique. Live-attenuated vaccines elicit powerful immune responses while inactivated vaccines provide immunization options to those that are immunocompromised. Both platforms of vaccines are a classic and proven technique used to protect against diseases. However, we must also remember that live-attenuated vaccines carry an inherent safety risk, more so than other vaccine platforms, and inactivated vaccines require more doses to protect against a disease. Both vaccine platforms are relatively expensive and time consuming to produce. We must consider these advantages and disadvantages when determining the best vaccine platform to use against COVID-19.

Chapter 8 - Recombinant Vaccines

By: Ivan Quan

Whereas inactivated or attenuated vaccines use the virus itself to stimulate antibody generation, vaccines with recombinant technology use only specific parts of viruses. Recall how phagocytes from the innate immune system will kill pathogens when detected in the body. Phagocytes will then present unique small parts of the pathogen to the adaptive immune system to help with identification. These identifying parts of viruses are proteins called antigens, sparking the adaptive immune system into action. Recombinant vaccines are designed to expose the body to the antigen, unaccompanied by the rest of the pathogen. After exposure, when the antibody is recognized by the body, the immune system will develop antibodies specific to the antigen, allowing it to keep memory of specific pathogens. These antibodies are a large aspect of humoral immunity, which refers to the immunological macromolecules circulating the body. After developing antibodies through the humoral response, the immune system will be able to quickly recognize and kill the pathogen in future encounters. Some recombinant vaccines also trigger the cell-mediated response, which is the immune system's approach to killing infected cells. Although different types of recombinant vaccines have different mechanisms to developing immunity, they are all made using recombinant DNA technology. This involves the joining of different DNA fragments, allowing scientists to configure DNA segments. As you might imagine, the versatility of this technology is considerable, reflected in its extensive use in biology.

Protein Subunit Vaccines

There are two general ways that recombinant vaccines can work. The traditional recombinant vaccine method involves producing massive quantities of antigen proteins outside the body, which will be injected during vaccine administration. To understand how these vaccines are made, we must understand how proteins are made. The central dogma of molecular biology states that information flows from DNA, to RNA, and finally, to proteins. A chef's recipe is a classic analogy describing this informational flow. A cookbook found in a library can represent the DNA stored in the nucleus. Recipes found in the cookbook are analogous to genes in the DNA. These recipes cannot be made directly into food, since you cannot cook in the library. Instead, you can copy down the recipe on a piece of paper to take to your kitchen. This process is known as transcription. Likewise, when DNA in the nucleus (a recipe in the cookbook) gets transcribed to RNA (transcribed notes on paper), it exits the nucleus, and enters the internal fluid of the cell known as the cytosol. After bringing the recipe to the kitchen, food can be made with the instructions you transcribed on paper. Correspondingly, inside the cellular cytosol, machinery known as ribosomes make proteins by following instructions found in the RNA through a process known as translation. Bacterial and viral pathogens both use proteins. Whereas bacteria have built-in transcriptional and translational machinery, viruses generally rely on the machinery of the host cell to reproduce. A key takeaway from this, is that the structure of proteins is encoded in DNA. Therefore, if we can acquire the DNA encoding the antigen, we can use transcription and translation machinery to mass-produce antigens. Additionally, entire protein genes are not usually necessary. In many cases, our immune system recognizes only a part, or a subunit of the protein as an antigen.

Recombinant DNA technology can be used to exploit the transcription and translation machinery in bacteria to make antigens. Bacteria have the capacity to ingest small circular fragments of DNA known as plasmids. Through a recombinant process, we can insert a gene encoding the pathogenic antigen protein subunit into a plasmid. This plasmid will then be inserted into a yeast cell, which acts as an antigen factory, continuing to multiply and produce large quantities of the protein. When a sufficient amount of antigen has been produced by the recombinant yeast bacteria, the protein can be extracted and purified to be used in a vaccine.

Recombinant protein subunit vaccines have several advantages over the more traditional live attenuated or inactivated vaccines. Although live attenuated vaccines can induce incredibly strong immune responses, many immunocompromised individuals are unable to safely take the vaccine. As subunit vaccines have no chance of bodily infection, they can be used by everyone. The risk of harmful side effects is also minimized, as the vaccine only includes the antigen subunit itself. Furthermore, recombinant protein subunit vaccines are generally more economical to produce at massive scale than both live attenuated and inactivated vaccines (M. Wang et al., 2016). However, because subunit vaccines do not typically elicit a strong cell-mediated response, they may often require multiple doses or an adjuvant, an addition to increase the effectiveness of the vaccine to maintain immunity (Vartak & Sucheck, 2016).

There are many attempts to develop a vaccine using this method, and it has the largest number of vaccine candidates for preventing SARS-CoV-2 infection. One of these candidates, named NVX-CoV2373, is being developed by the American company Novavax. Using recombinant DNA technology, Novavax has produced antigens derived from the SARS-CoV-2 spike protein. In the same way that SARS-CoV-2 binds to receptors in the body, preclinical trials have demonstrated that the developed protein binds similarly to receptors (Tian et al., 2020). This shows that the structure of NVX-CoV2373 is congruent with the structure of the viral protein, allowing the antibodies generated in response to NVX-CoV2373 to work against the virus. In addition to the antigen, the vaccine will also contain Novavax's proprietary Matrix-M adjuvant. Matrix-M has been shown to heighten the immune response of other Novavax vaccines such as the seasonal influenza vaccine, and it is therefore also added to their COVID-19 vaccine (Magnusson et al., 2018). Currently, the vaccine is undergoing phase I trials, with human testing on participants in Australia, and with plans to move into phase II and III testing shortly after.

Adenovirus Vector Vaccines

Another more experimental approach to developing a recombinant vaccine has recently been brought to light, and is currently seeing great potential in protection against SARS-CoV-2. Adenovirus vector vaccines, as they are called, are currently one of the frontrunners in the race to COVID-19 vaccine development. An adenovirus refers to a certain family of DNA viruses causing a wide range of illnesses. This method works on the basis of using a modified DNA adenovirus as a vehicle to deliver antigen proteins. Viruses have the ability to hijack cell resources, forcing cells to make viral proteins. By exploiting this, scientists have engineered viruses that are capable of manufacturing any antigen of choice.

First, viruses must be modified such that they are no longer able to reproduce. Certain genes responsible for replication are inactivated, which eliminates any chance of infection. The deletion of the replication sequences also makes room to insert a gene of choice. For vaccines, DNA encoding an antigen would be added via recombinant DNA processes. Adenoviruses in particular are used as vectors for vaccines, because they work well under genetic manipulation. Additionally, adenoviruses generally infect a wide range of cells in the body, allowing it to spread the vaccine more effectively (Khanal et al., 2018). After the antigen DNA is inserted into viruses, the vaccine is ready to be used. The vaccine works by having the modified adenovirus infect body cells after injection. However, the virus will not replicate and grow like a normal virus would. Instead, it starts to induce the infected host cell to express the inserted gene, which in the case of a vaccine, is the antigen.

As the antigen is produced by the host cells, it is presented to the adaptive immune system, readying the body for defending against the target virus in the future.

Adenovirus vector based vaccines provide numerous advantages over conventional vaccine types. Whereas recombinant protein subunit vaccines merely activate the creation of antibodies by triggering the humoral response, adenovirus vector vaccines also activate the cell-mediated response. In reaction to being infected with the adenovirus, cytotoxic T cells will spring into action to kill the infected cells (Ura et al., 2014). Similar to the reason why live attenuated vaccines provide more effective protection than inactivated vaccines, adenovirus vector based vaccines administer stronger protection than protein subunit vaccines. The closer the vaccine can get to a real infection event, the better the immune response is to the vaccine. It then follows that a better immune response leads to better immunological memory of the antigen, which results in a stronger defence against the pathogen in the future (Ura et al., 2014). The effectiveness of adenovirus vector based vaccines is evident, in that it is able to simulate a real infection event without putting the patient in danger of an infection.

In the midst of the pandemic, adenovirus vector based vaccines make up some of the vaccines furthest along the line of testing and development. AZD1222 (formerly known as ChAdOx1 nCoV-19) is a vaccine candidate developed by the University of Oxford using adenovirus vector technology. The vaccine is based on the chimpanzee common cold virus, modified to prevent the virus's reproduction. When injected, the modified adenovirus will infect cells and cause them to produce the SARS-CoV-2 antigen. This was accomplished by inserting the DNA encoding this protein into the viral genome. This triggers both a cell-mediated response as a result of an adenovirus infection in the host cells and a humoral response from the detection of antigens in the body. Overall, this builds up the adaptive immune system to be prepared for a SARS-CoV-2 infection. In preclinical studies, the effectiveness of AZD1222 has been tested on rhesus monkeys. When administered a single shot of the vaccine, the humoral and cell-mediated responses were observed as expected. Twenty-eight days after vaccination, all monkeys developed antibodies against the virus. At this time, the vaccinated monkeys were also introduced to the SARS-CoV-2 virus in a challenge trial. Compared to non-vaccinated animals, the respiratory tracts of vaccinated monkeys had significantly less viruses detected. Furthermore, the vaccinated rhesus monkeys did not develop pneumonia and thus, had no lung damage (Doremalen et al., 2020b). Though these tests demonstrate the impressive protective effectiveness of the vaccine, its effectiveness in social immunity is uncertain. Although the vaccine was found to protect monkeys against disease, this study also found that SARS-CoV-2 viral RNA was detected in the nose with the same quantity as the unvaccinated monkeys. This is a sign that the virus was still able to multiply, even though it did not cause disease. Since the virus still existed in the respiratory system of the vaccinated monkeys, it is possible that it could still be transmitted, diminishing the chance of attaining herd immunity through this vaccine. Like many other vaccines in development during the pandemic, AZD1222 undergoes combined clinical trials. Results from phase I/II testing indicated no severe adverse events, and antibody production was observed (Folegatti et al., 2020b). Phase II/III testing is underway with thousands of participants volunteering to receive doses of the vaccine candidate. Although still in trial, Sarah Gilbert, Professor of Vaccinology at the University of Oxford, commented on the clinical trials: "We're very happy that we're seeing the right sort of immune response that will give protection, and not the wrong sort." Hinting towards optimism, Oxford gives hope towards developing a functional SARS-CoV-2 vaccine.

The Chinese company CanSino Biologics has also made an adenovirus vector based vaccine for COVID-19, named Ad5-nCoV. Like AZD1222, the inserted gene encodes the SARS-CoV-2 spike protein. However, while the vector in AZD1222 is a modified chimpanzee common cold virus, the Ad5-nCoV vector is based on a human common cold virus. An obstacle that must be overcome when using human adenoviruses as vectors, is that people who have been previously infected with the adenovirus would have antibodies defending them against the vector. If a person has been previously exposed to this specific strain of common cold, it is possible that their immune system, being already primed to attack this threat, would kill the adenovirus vector before it gets the chance to release its DNA that encodes the desired antigens (Tomita et al., 2012). These pre-existing neutralizing antibodies could render the vaccine ineffective in a subset of the population. Since animal adenoviruses, like the vector used in AZD1222 do not widely spread to humans, neutralizing antibodies are not of concern. In the Ad5-nCoV phase I clinical trial, it was shown that the vaccine was safe and produced an immune response in both people with pre-existing neutralizing antibodies, and without. However, those with pre-existing neutralizing antibodies had a slower and weaker peak immune response to the vaccine, which could impact its effectiveness (Zhu et al., 2020). As soon as it was deemed to be safe, and to some extent effective, it was approved to be used in the Chinese military. As of July 2020, CanSino is taking next steps towards development, having already initiated phase II clinical trials. Plans also exist to move Ad5-nCoV to phase III of clinical trials in the near future.

Overall, the different types of recombinant vaccines aim to expose the body to an antigen, rather than the whole pathogen, to trigger an immune response with the goal of future protection against the pathogen. The more traditional protein subunit vaccine uses recombinant DNA technology to produce parts of proteins to be administered as a vaccine, while adenovirus vector based vaccines use recombinant DNA technology to insert a pathogenic protein gene into a modified adenovirus. As both have their pros and cons, a multitude of recombinant vaccines are in development with the goal of preventing COVID-19. As adenovirus vector vaccines are still quite experimental, the candidates that are developed to fight COVID-19 will certainly pave the way for the future vaccines using this technology.

Chapter 9 - Nucleic Acid Vaccines

By: Ivy Quan

Immune Response

Nucleic acid vaccines are composed of DNA or RNA segments that encode a viral antigen of choice. Both DNA and RNA store genetic information; in this case, they store sequences that can create proteins found on certain pathogens (C. Zhang et al., 2019). On a general level, nucleic acid vaccines stimulate the immune system in a similar way to adenovirus vector vaccines or recombinant subunit vaccines. They expose the body to the antigens of a particular pathogen, allowing the immune system to produce and store specific antibodies. However, nucleic acid vaccines differ in a few key ways. Recall that information flows from DNA to mRNA, to proteins. If we revisit the central dogma analogy to cooking that was mentioned in the previous chapter, DNA vaccines function by adding another cookbook into your host cell's library, while mRNA vaccines give recipes to your host cell's kitchen directly. DNA vaccines encoding for a viral antigen must enter the host cell's nucleus where host cell machinery will use it as a template to produce mRNA. The mRNA will then exit the nucleus where other enzymes can use it to produce proteins. In vaccines, these proteins will be antigens - the identification tags for specific pathogens that can trigger an immune response. RNA vaccines are simply strands of mRNA encoding the antigen, and therefore are ready to take advantage of host cell machinery to produce antigenic proteins upon entering our cells.

Once the proteins are produced within the host cell, they can follow two distinct pathways. Some antigens will exit the cell and will act in a similar fashion to recombinant subunit vaccines (C. Zhang et al., 2019). However, nucleic acid vaccines can elicit stronger immune responses than subunit vaccines because they use host cells as large antigen factories, whereas subunit vaccines only provide a set amount of antigens per dosage. These viral proteins will circulate the body until they encounter a phagocyte that will engulf the antigen. Phagocytes will digest and present a portion of the proteins to the T cells of the acquired immune system. This activates the acquired immune system which produces and stores specific antibodies. The acquired immune response also involves killer T cells that kill infected cells. This is where the other antigen pathway comes into play. Viral proteins from nucleic acid vaccines can also be placed on special receptors on the outside of the host cell. Stuck to the outside of the cell, these proteins act as beacons to alert killer T cells that the host cell is "infected". Of course, the nucleic acid vaccines do not actually infect host cells as a typical virus would, but they stimulate the cell-mediated response from killer T cells nonetheless. Through these two pathways, both DNA and RNA vaccines can effectively elicit humoral and cell-mediated responses (C. Zhang et al., 2019).

DNA Vaccines

Part of the reason why nucleic acid vaccines garnered attention during the COVID-19 pandemic is because of their many advantages over traditional attenuated, inactivated, and recombinant vaccines. Live attenuated vaccines require chicken eggs to produce and inactivated vaccines require cultivating many viruses to kill for use in the vaccine. Meanwhile, the production of DNA vaccines is similar to that of recombinant subunit vaccines. DNA encoding an antigen is placed inside plasmids, which are circular DNA strands from bacteria, and are then injected into yeast cells. When the yeast cells divide and grow, they will also replicate the DNA plasmid of interest. After several generations, the DNA plasmids can be isolated from their cells and can be used as the active ingredient of the vaccine (Khan, 2013). This makes production of DNA vaccines faster and cheaper than traditional live attenuated or inactivated vaccines. DNA vaccines are also safer than traditional vaccines in production and immunization because the production process does not involve cultivating dangerous pathogens. In addition, DNA vaccines have no chance of infection since they are only carriers of genetic information for a single protein. In these ways, DNA vaccines and recombinant subunit vaccines have a lot of common advantages. However, unlike subunit vaccines, DNA vaccines can induce both a cell-mediated and humoral immune response. Moreover, one of the major benefits unique to DNA vaccines is their stability under different temperatures (Khan, 2013). Traditional vaccines require cold storage which makes transportation and storage in remote or developing nations extremely challenging. The stability of DNA makes the transport and storage of DNA vaccines easier and less expensive.

However, DNA vaccines also have some notable disadvantages. Although effective in small lab animals such as rats, so far DNA vaccines have not been able to produce strong immune responses in larger animals such as sheep or humans. As such, the only licensed DNA vaccines as of 2020 are for animals, which include a canine and feline vaccine against rabies (Redding & Werner, 2009). Their relatively low immunogenicity may be because the DNA must overcome many barriers to be effective. DNA vaccines must pass through the cell membrane as well as the nuclear membrane prior to its arrival in the nucleus, where it can then take advantage of the host cell machinery. Only approximately 0.1% of the injected DNA will end up in the nucleus, which results in its low vaccine potency (Lechardeur et al., 1999). To address this issue, researchers have developed electroporation as a vaccination strategy. Electroporation involves applying pulses of electricity to the injection site after vaccination. This causes temporary pores to form on the membranes of cells at the injection site, enhancing the ability of cells to take in the DNA vaccine by 10-1000 fold (Sardesai & Weiner, 2011). Electroporation, among other emerging enhancement technologies, improves the strength of the immune response elicited by DNA vaccines, and could be integral in the development of a successful COVID-19 vaccine candidate.

The frontrunner for DNA vaccine candidates against COVID-19 is Inovio's INO-4800 vaccine delivered by electroporation. Inovio is a DNA medicine company, and their DNA vaccine candidate INO-4800 codes for the SARS-CoV-2 spike protein. In its preclinical and phase I trials, INO-4800 produced promising results. The preclinical trials involved subjecting mice to a challenge trial, in which the immunized mice did not show any viral replication in their lungs. In phase I clinical trials, 34 of 36 human participants demonstrated both humoral and cell-mediated immune responses with only mild side effects such as redness at the injection site ("INOVIO announces positive", 2020). With these promising interim results, Inovio plans to proceed with combined phase II/III trials to further examine efficacy in August of 2020.

RNA Vaccines

RNA vaccines also have many advantages over traditional vaccines. Like DNA vaccines, they do not pose risk of infection, they can stimulate both humoral and cell-mediated immune responses, and they have a quicker manufacturing process. However, RNA vaccines can be produced even more quickly and more effectively than DNA vaccines via egg-free and cell-free processes. Using a DNA template encoding the antigen, manufacturers can mass produce mRNA strands with enzymes in solution to catalyze multiple reactions (C. Zhang et al., 2019). The lack of eggs or cells makes the production of RNA vaccines less expensive and much quicker - two traits which are highly beneficial to the development of any vaccine candidate, especially during a global pandemic. The nature of mRNA vaccine production also allows the vaccine to be customizable; the same enzymes and processes can be used to produce any mRNA sequence. Since all proteins can be encoded in mRNA, manufacturers can theoretically make a vaccine for any pathogen or toxin if the genetic sequence of the antigen is known. Once this technology is refined, the development of RNA vaccines could shorten the time between the onset of an epidemic or pandemic and the distribution of nation-wide vaccine programs.

If there are so many benefits to RNA vaccines, a valid question to ask is: why aren't there any mRNA vaccines on the market today? Although this technology has already shown plenty of potential, it is still relatively new. One major setback for RNA vaccines is their instability within a human host. Floating around our body are natural enzymes that degrade mRNA (Liu, 2019). We can compare this to a situation in which all the recipes are destroyed before they make it to the kitchen. As a result, more attention was put into DNA vaccine development instead of RNA vaccines (Liu, 2019). However, due to several advancements in RNA stabilizing technology, there is newfound excitement amongst researchers. Lipid nanoparticle (LNP) capsules for the mRNA are one of the technological advancements. LNP capsules act as a spherical shield that protects mRNA strands from being degraded by enzymes and increases the efficiency of mRNA vaccines (Blakney et al., 2019). LNPs are popular delivery mechanisms for manufacturers attempting to develop a mRNA vaccine for COVID-19.

The two trailblazers for mRNA vaccine development for COVID-19 are Moderna and BioNTech/Pfizer. Both the mRNA-1273 candidate by Moderna and the BNT162 candidate by BioNtech/Pfizer are LNP encapsulated mRNA vaccines that code for the SARS-CoV-2 spike protein, and both have shown promising results. In the phase I trials for mRNA-1273, all 45 participants demonstrated humoral and cell-mediated immune responses with no serious adverse events. Antibody levels in participants vaccinated with mRNA-1273 were higher than the typical antibody levels in people who recovered from COVID-19, demonstrating an efficacious vaccine (Jackson et al., 2020). Preliminary data from the phase I/II trial of BNT162 also looked promising. All 60 participants demonstrated high antibody levels and a majority of participants who received booster shots also demonstrated cell-mediated immune responses. Amongst all participants, there were no severe adverse events and mild adverse effects were tolerable ("Pfizer and BioNTech announce", 2020). Moderna and BioNtech/Pfizer expect to begin their phase III and II/III trials respectively in the late summer of 2020.

Aside from the conventional mRNA vaccine candidates being developed by Moderna and BioNtech/Pfizer, researchers have developed another subtype of mRNA vaccines named self-amplifying mRNA. While the conventional mRNA vaccines only encode the antigen, self-amplifying mRNA also encodes for an RNA replication enzyme, a viral protein that replicates mRNA (C. Zhang et al., 2019). The RNA replication enzyme helps viruses make many strands of mRNA from a single strand so viruses can multiply. We can take advantage of the RNA replication enzyme by using it to increase the efficacy of mRNA vaccines. If we revisit our cooking analogy in which we compared mRNA to recipes in a kitchen, this replication enzyme is analogous to a photocopier. The photocopier can make more copies of the recipes so that more chefs can make more food. As such, having an mRNA strand that encodes for both an antigen and an RNA replication enzyme will increase the efficacy of an RNA vaccine. Essentially, a lower dosage of a self-amplifying RNA vaccine can elicit the same quality of immune response as a higher dosage of a conventional RNA vaccine.

A vaccine candidate for COVID-19 using self-amplifying RNA technology is COVAC1 by Imperial College London. COVAC1 is an LNP-encapsulated self-amplifying mRNA vaccine that encodes for the SARS-CoV-2 spike protein. In preclinical trials with very promising results, researchers immunized mice and compared their immune responses to human patients who had recovered from COVID-19. They found that the RNA vaccine was able to stimulate the production of antibodies in mice that neutralized SARS-CoV-2. Even the lowest doses of the vaccine resulted in higher levels of antibodies in mice than the antibody levels found in recovered COVID-19 patients (McKay et al., 2020). These preclinical results suggest that COVAC1 can stimulate a sufficiently strong immune response to be effective in preventing COVID-19. In July 2020, COVAC1 commenced combined phase I/II trials involving 300 participants (O'Hare & Wighton, 2020). Professor Robin Shattock, Principal Investigator in COVAC1's trials, shared his optimism during an interview with The Guardian: "I'm cautiously optimistic that it will work as well as anything else that is being developed because it induces good immune responses in animal models, and we predict it will be the same in humans and it will be very safe because we are using such low doses," (Boseley, 2020a). As the first self-amplifying RNA vaccine to be tested on humans, these COVAC1 trials will pave the road for evolving nucleic acid vaccine technologies.

To recap, nucleic acid vaccines are made of either DNA or RNA encoding for an antigen. These DNA and RNA strands expose the body to antigens and stimulate both the humoral and cell-mediated immune responses by using host cells as antigen factories. Nucleic acid vaccines also offer unique advantages. Since DNA is stable at room temperature, DNA vaccines can be transported and stored for lengths of time without cold-storage, which would allow for immunization in areas without proper cooling equipment. On the other hand, RNA vaccines are incredibly quick to produce. Within 14 days of knowing the genomic code for SARS-CoV-2, Professor Robert Shattock and his team at Imperial College London synthesized a vaccine candidate ready for preclinical trials. In Professor Shattock's own words, his team went from, "code to candidate" in a matter of two weeks (O'Hare & Wighton, 2020). This unprecedented speed demonstrates the potential that RNA vaccines have to revolutionize the development of vaccines and how we respond to epidemics or pandemics. Since there have been no licensed nucleic acid vaccines for humans prior to the COVID-19 pandemic, the development and testing of these candidates against COVID-19 will undoubtedly advance our understanding of the efficacy and safety of nucleic acid vaccines in humans.

Chapter 10 - Convalescent Plasma Therapy

By: Evangelea Touliopoulos

As of July 2020, there is currently no approved vaccine available to provide immunity from COVID-19. However, the virus is still spreading through communities and forcing many additional safety measures, such as the cancellation of large events, the need to wear a facemask in public buildings, and the restructuring of workplaces and schools. Even with all these preventative measures, many people are still contracting the virus and becoming very sick. While society waits for the development of a vaccine, many other treatments are being explored to try and lessen some of the virus's symptoms and to help those who have COVID-19 make a speedy recovery. In this chapter, we are going to explore some of these treatments that are being used while society waits for a successful vaccine to be approved.

COVID-19 Convalescent Plasma Therapy

One potential treatment to help patients survive an infection from the SARS-CoV-2 virus is convalescent plasma therapy. This treatment works by having a patient who has recovered from a COVID-19 infection donate some of their plasma to transfuse into another patient who is currently suffering from COVID-19 and is displaying severe symptoms (Rajendran et al., 2020). Plasma is the clear, liquid part of the blood that remains after all the cellular components of blood are removed (Stanford Children's Health, n.d.). Cellular components of blood include red blood cells, white blood cells, and platelets (Stanford Children's Health, n.d.). The important thing about plasma with respect to convalescent plasma therapy is that it contains antibodies. Recall from earlier chapters that an antibody is a protein that is produced in response to pathogen exposure, and provides immunity to that pathogen (National Cancer Institute, 2011). One important thing to recognize is that after fighting off an invader, patients will have developed humoral immunity to that pathogen. This means that their blood plasma will have very high levels of antibodies targeting that specific pathogen. Thus, a patient who recently recovered from COVID-19 will have a lot of SARS-CoV-2 antibodies in their plasma. By transfusing the plasma of the recovered COVID-19 patient into the patient sick with COVID-19, the sick patient will acquire the COVID-19 antibodies of the recovered patient (Rajendran et al., 2020). These antibodies will theoretically help the sick patient clear the pathogen from their system and recover from COVID-19 (Rajendran et al., 2020). This treatment is most effective when it is administered shortly after the onset of symptoms, or within 14 days of infection (Brown & McCullough, 2020). The protection from the virus given by convalescent plasma therapy can last from weeks to months, depending on the health and immune system of the patient (Brown & McCullough, 2020).

While convalescent plasma therapy is not a vaccine, as it does not provide preventative protection from infection, many consider it to be a form of passive immunization (Marano et al., 2016). This is because it grants a person immediate short term immunity to the virus through the transfusion of antibodies (Marano et al., 2016). To compare a vaccine would expose the body to the virus so that it can build up its own antibodies, however, convalescent plasma therapy involves transfusing already developed antibodies specific to the virus into a patient. There has been evidence of convalescent plasma therapy working for the treatment of other pathogens. For instance, there have been trials that show that convalescent plasma therapy works on viruses such as measles and SARS-CoV (Brown & McCullough, 2020). While many of the clinical trials on SARS-CoV convalescent plasma therapy were disbanded once the threat of SARS-CoV receded, there is enough evidence to show that convalescent plasma therapy can be helpful in treating SARS-CoV, a virus that is very similar to SARS-CoV-2 (Brown & McCullough, 2020). These promising results have encouraged researchers to investigate further into the usage of convalescent plasma therapy to treat COVID-19.

Effect of Convalescent Plasma Therapy on COVID-19

The first thing that needs to be considered when g using convalescent plasma therapy to treat a pathogen is the question of where the convalescent plasma is going to come from. Recovered COVID-19 patients who meet the eligibility criteria for a blood transfusion would undergo apheresis (Tiberghien et al., n.d.). Apheresis is a form of blood donation where the blood is extracted from the body, the plasma is removed from the blood, and then the remainder of the blood cells are reinserted back into the body (BC Children's Hospital, n.d.). This technique allows more plasma to be collected than in a regular blood donation and protects the patient from feeling the side effects of blood donation as acutely, since virtually none of the red blood cells are extracted from the body (Tiberghien et al., n.d.). Apheresis should be done within four months of recovery from COVID-19, as that is when the relevant antibodies will be the most abundant in the blood (Tiberghien et al., n.d.). The extracted plasma should also be tested to ensure that it has a sufficient level of antibodies because the levels of antibodies in those recovered from COVID-19 may vary from person to person (Tiberghien et al., n.d.). Finally, some experts say that the plasma should also be tested for the presence of viral RNA because there is a possibility that the virus could still be present even when the patient is asymptomatic (Tiberghien et al., n.d.). If there were to be viral RNA in the plasma, there would be the possibility of transfusion-transmitted COVID-19 (Tiberghien et al., n.d.). However, this screening is more of a precautionary measure, as it is not expected for the pathogen to be present in the majority of the convalescent plasma donations, and transmission of a respiratory virus through blood transfusion has never before been reported (Tiberghien et al., n.d.).

Once the convalescent plasma with a sufficient amount of antibodies is acquired, the therapy is ready to be administered to sick patients. The most effective way of using convalescent plasma therapy on patients who have COVID-19 is either as a form of prophylaxis, which means administering the therapy before the onset of symptoms as a way to prevent illness, or as a therapeutic, when the plasma therapy is administered shortly after symptoms begin (Tiberghien et al., n.d.). If convalescent plasma therapy is administered after the patients exhibit severe symptoms, such as systemic organ failure, there is a chance that the therapy will not reduce the negative symptoms of the virus or help the body clear of the virus (Tiberghien et al., n.d.). However, this does not mean that convalescent plasma therapy should be ignored completely as an option for patients who have developed severe symptoms of COVID-19 (Tiberghien et al., n.d.). In a study conducted in China during 2020, five critically ill patients who had all developed acute respiratory distress syndrome and were on mechanical ventilators were administered neutralizing antibodies through convalescent plasma (Tiberghien et al., n.d.). All five of these patients had an improved clinical outcome after the use of convalescent plasma therapy (Tiberghien et al., n.d.). This demonstrates how the therapy still has potential, even if it is not optimal, when it is administered later after severe symptoms of the virus appear.

Another promising aspect of convalescent plasma therapy is that there have not been any severe adverse effects when it is administered to COVID-19 patients (Tiberghien et al., n.d.). There have been a couple of instances of an increase in temperature, itching, or skin rashes, but nothing life-threatening (Tiberghien et al., n.d.). This is the expected outcome as human convalescent plasma transfers are commonplace procedures in hospitals (Bloch et al., 2020). The only difference between convalescent plasma therapy to treat COVID-19 and a routine convalescent plasma transfer is that the former contains COVID-19 antibodies while the latter does not, which should not affect the safety of the therapy.

Another positive sign is that there have been multiple studies about the use of COVID-19 convalescent plasma on critically ill patients that have yielded positive results. A study conducted by the University of Iowa Hospitals and Clinics confirmed that the majority of potential plasma donors tested had plasma that was rich with COVID-19 antibodies (Knudson & Jackson, 2020). However, as expected, there was a significant variation in antibody levels amongst the potential donors and several donors were rendered ineligible because they had insufficient antibody levels (Knudson & Jackson, 2020). This study also found that if the plasma was being taken too soon after recovery from COVID-19, there was a small chance that it would still contain viral RNA, which means they would be ineligible for donation as this could introduce more of the virus into the transfusion recipient (Knudson & Jackson, 2020). Although there was little former evidence that suggests viral RNA would pose a challenge, this study demonstrates the need to screen for the possibility that plasma could contain viral RNA.

There are a variety of other ongoing clinical studies about convalescent plasma therapy to treat COVID-19. Overall, most demonstrate that convalescent plasma therapy lowers mortality and has very few adverse effects (Valk et al., 2020). However, many researchers are pointing out the need for more comprehensive clinical trials for convalescent plasma therapy as there are very few guidelines for how it should be administered. For example, what is the optimal amount of antibodies that a patient should receive for them to recover? How many times should a patient be injected with antibodies? When is the optimal time to collect antibodies from the donor? Furthermore, many researchers are arguing that since the clinical trials being performed are very small and are mostly not randomized, it is hard to draw definitive conclusions about convalescent plasma therapy for COVID-19. So even though it seems highly probable that convalescent plasma therapy has therapeutic effects on patients infected with COVID-19, researchers still do not have a definitive answer.

Moral Questions Concerning Convalescent Plasma Therapy

So far, COVID-19 convalescent plasma therapy has been approved for patients who have been hospitalized due to severe cases of COVID-19 in many places around the world, including Canada and the United States. However, many people are questioning whether it should be approved for different groups of people as well. For example, should convalescent plasma therapy be administered to people who have not yet been infected with the virus, but are considered a high-risk population? Some examples of potential high-risk populations would be seniors and healthcare workers. While this treatment would not be as effective as a successful vaccine, convalescent plasma therapy could still reduce these high-risk groups' likelihood of contracting COVID-19 or it could reduce the severity of their symptoms should they get sick. However, as there is not nearly enough COVID-19 convalescent plasma available to provide everyone with a transfusion, how would it be decided who would get this preventative therapy? Furthermore, what about people who are already sick with the virus but have yet to present with severe symptoms? Giving them COVID-19 convalescent plasma would reduce the likelihood that they develop severe, life-threatening symptoms. However, there is also the possibility that they would not have developed severe symptoms anyways. In this case, one could argue that the plasma would have been more useful had it been administered to someone else.

Another ethical concern is about obtaining the COVID-19 convalescent plasma. Right now, it is obtained entirely from voluntary donations by those who have recovered from COVID-19 and who are eligible for blood donation. However, as there is such a high demand for the plasma throughout the

COVID-19 pandemic, would it be ethical to incentivize people to donate their plasma with monetary rewards? Considering that having a larger supply would likely correlate with saving more lives, it seems like this could be worth the money. But, where would the money that is being used to incentivize the donors come from? Some options would be the patients receiving the treatment, the government, or a third party organization, which all present their own ethical concerns.

Evidently, there are many important questions to consider about how COVID-19 convalescent plasma therapy should be administered and collected so that it will save the most lives while operating in a fair and equitable manner.

Big Picture on COVID-19 Convalescent Plasma Therapy

So far, there is some evidence to suggest that COVID-19 convalescent plasma therapy is able to reduce the mortality rate of patients hospitalized with severe symptoms of COVID-19. It also has been found that recently recovered COVID-19 patients are usually good candidates for convalescent plasma donations. While more research is needed on the ideal way COVID-19 convalescent plasma therapy should be conducted, and more importantly, if COVID-19 convalescent plasma therapy is actually as effective as it is hypothesized to be, it is still a highly valuable potential treatment for COVID-19. Considering that historically, convalescent plasma therapy was used as a way to prevent illnesses before the development of vaccines, it is only logical that it could be of great use to communities impacted by COVID-19 while a vaccine is being developed. The passive immunity provided by the convalescent plasma therapy could save many lives and help in the fight against the SARS-CoV-2 virus.

Chapter 11 - Barriers to COVID-19 Vaccine Development

By: Ivan Quan

Previously, we have mentioned how a vast majority of vaccine candidates do not make it to market. Usually, this is due to an inadequate immune response triggered by the vaccine. These shortcomings are hurdles that developing vaccines must overcome, including potential COVID-19 vaccines. To understand the barriers that may cause COVID-19 vaccines to fail, we must first understand what vaccine failure means. There is no vaccine that is 100% effective, so a vaccine that is less than 100% effective does not indicate defect (World Health Organization, 2013). Regardless of the type of vaccine or the pathogen targeted, not everyone who takes the vaccine will gain immunity. As such, vaccine failure refers to when a person is susceptible to contracting a disease, despite being vaccinated against it. If a vaccine candidate fails to the extent that communities given the vaccine are not protected, it will not pass clinical trials. Although many instances of vaccine failure can be attributed to logistical issues such as improper vaccine use, improper handling, or expiry due to a finite shelf life, this chapter will mainly focus on technical reasons that vaccines may fail.

Primary Vaccine Failure

Primary vaccine failure occurs when a vaccine either does not induce antibody production, or does not produce enough antibodies to defend against the pathogen (Hinman et al., 1992). One reason that primary failure may occur is due to a host-related issue. Different populations, with variables including age, immune health, and genetics can experience different immune responses to the same vaccine. The ideal dosage for each age range is determined in clinical testing, where researchers optimize for effective antibody response while minimizing the adverse effects. However, there are cases where a vaccine is unable to induce antibody expression in a portion of certain demographics. Usually, it is in a portion of youth and the elderly where vaccines may not work as well. This is an issue that many vaccines, including COVID-19 vaccine candidates, must face. Because vaccines work by triggering an immune response to generate antibodies, older people with weaker immune systems will not react as strongly to vaccines. A smaller quantity of antibodies will be generated, resulting in a potentially weaker protection against future encounters with the pathogen. Although many vaccines, including the influenza vaccine, counteract this by increasing the dosage as much as four-fold in the elderly, testing must be done in clinical trials to determine whether an increased dosage is safe and efficacious (J. Wang et al., 2016). Considering that the elderly are the most vulnerable to the COVID-19 disease, it is of utmost importance that they receive protection. However, if we discover that a vaccine is not efficacious in the elderly, they can still be protected through herd immunity. While a vulnerable person may not have antibodies against the pathogen, the pathogen would have little opportunity to spread to the elderly if everyone in contact with them has immunity. However, with some vaccines, herd immunity is not possible. Even in completely healthy individuals, primary vaccine failure can occur, with some vaccines more susceptible to failure than others. For instance, up to 10% of healthy individuals given the hepatitis B vaccine do not produce an adequate level of antibodies to protect them against the pathogen (Wiedermann et al., 2016). Though this is likely due to a genetic predisposition, it does not predict that the same individual would be less protected by other vaccines (Garner-Spitzer et al., 2013). If enough of the population is nonresponsive to a vaccine, herd immunity, which relies on a high percentage of the community being immune, may diminish. Through simulated population models, researchers have determined that vaccine efficacy must be greater than 60% for COVID-19 herd immunity to be effective if everyone receives the vaccine. This efficacy threshold rises to 80% as vaccine coverage drops to 60% (Bartsch et al., 2020). Though this highlights the importance of widespread vaccine distribution, it also emphasizes the need for high efficacy. So far, vaccine candidates show promising results in terms of efficacy. With a sample size in the tens, both Oxford's phase I/II trial on AZD1222, as well as Moderna's phase I trial on mRNA-1273 showed sufficient antibody development in all participants (Folegatti et al., 2020b; Jackson et al., 2020). Though these results may be reassuring, there is more to COVID-19 protection than short-term antibody response, as we will discover when discussing secondary vaccine failure.

Antibody-Dependent Enhancement of Disease

Another instance of primary failure is antibody-dependent enhancement of disease (ADE), which has received much attention in the immunological community due to signs of its presence in SARS-CoV-2. Although this seems paradoxical, in a subset of viral diseases, the development of antibodies may actually cause the disease to worsen. Recall how viruses have proteins on their surface that bind to cellular receptors as a path of entry into a cell, resulting in infection. If an antibody is present, it will bind to the viral protein, which both prevents it from entering and infecting cells, and marks it to be engulfed by macrophages of the immune system. As macrophages have surface receptors that bind to antibodies, a typical virus marked with an antibody will bind to the macrophage receptor. The macrophage will then engulf and digest the virus. However, in the case of ADE, the virus may infect the macrophage after being engulfed (Halstead et al., 2010). Rather than being digested, the virus uses the macrophage's antibody receptors as a way to enter the cell, and exploits the macrophage's cell machinery to reproduce, causing further infection. In most cases, ADE is only a concern when an antibody binds suboptimally to the virus. Suboptimal binding can happen when the antigen present on the virus has a slightly dissimilar structure to the antigen that the antibody was initially made for (Iwasaki & Yang, 2020). This structural variation is often attributed to small genetic differences between similar virus strains, or a high mutation rate of the antigen.

As ADE has been found to occur in the family of coronaviruses, it is a potential barrier that vaccines developed for COVID-19 may have to overcome. It is crucial to note that ADE is exceedingly rare, and has only been linked to a handful of viral species at most. Although it is imperative to emphasize this risk when investigating vaccines against COVID-19, it is just as important to keep in mind that a licensed vaccine that has passed clinical testing will not induce ADE. Historically, ADE has proven to be a challenge in the development of MERS and SARS vaccines (Liang et al., 2020). Animal studies have shown that after developing antibodies against SARS, reexposure to the pathogen resulted in viral infection of macrophages. Although the exact mechanism is still unknown, researchers hypothesize that antibodies targeting the spike protein gave the virus a path of entry inside macrophages (Wan et al., 2019). Recall how the receptor binding domain (RBD) is the part of the coronavirus spike protein that attaches to cellular receptors. When analyzing coronaviruses, the RBD was found to have a high rate of mutation, and is therefore slightly variable in structure. This variability in the RBD could contribute to suboptimal binding of antigens, which in turn, may cause ADE and the infection of macrophages (Ricke & Malone, 2020). Since a majority of COVID-19 vaccines in development target the spike protein, ADE could pose a serious threat to the success of a vaccine. In SARS, antibody concentration has also been linked to ADE. Whereas a high concentration successfully neutralized a SARS infection, lower concentrations of the antibody induced cell death in isolated cell cultures.

Much of the relationship between the immune response to SARS-CoV-2 and the risk of ADE is still relatively unknown. This hinders our ability to develop a vaccine perfectly suited to avoiding ADE altogether. As such, the testing of many vaccine approaches is our best way to find an effective vaccine that does not induce ADE. Since the vaccine platform, protein target, dosage administered, and dosing schedule are all aspects of vaccines that influence antibody response, evaluating these factors can give insight on the prevalence of ADE in vaccine candidates. The preferred testing method of ADE is an animal challenge study. After vaccinating animals, we can test the effectiveness of the generated antibodies by reexposing them to the virus and judging their condition. As we have seen in the past with SARS-CoV vaccine development, even in the face of possible ADE, vaccine efficacy is entirely possible (Qin et al., 2006). Although it is unclear as to why certain vaccines are able to circumvent ADE, the simple fact that many have this quality gives optimism. This sentiment is also reflected in several SARS-CoV-2 candidates. ADE was not observed when testing Sinovac's CoronaVac inactivated vaccine, even when antibody concentrations were low (Gao et al., 2020).

Interestingly, ADE may be a factor contributing to COVID-19's deadliness in the elderly population, causing the disease to progress from relatively mild to highly severe. For a younger person, antibodies are likely developed quickly enough to eradicate the virus before it mutates excessively. As the immune system deteriorates in older populations, antibodies are produced slower, and in less quantity than in healthy youth and adults (Montecino-Rodriguez et al., 2013). While this does not affect the quality of antibodies produced, by the time a sufficient quantity of antibodies are produced to effectively combat SARS-CoV-2, the virus may have already mutated. These mutations could affect the structure of viral proteins, and in turn, cause unstable antigen binding which escalates the risk of ADE.

Secondary Vaccine Failure

In the case of secondary vaccine failure, protection from the pathogen is initially present, but fades substantially over time. However, waning quantities of antibodies are not a problem for some vaccines. Many individuals who have taken the measles vaccine experience a decline in antibody concentration to nearly undetectable levels after many years. Yet, upon reexposure to the virus, immunological memory quickly recognizes and responds to the antigen, massively boosting antibody levels (Krugman, 1983). For other vaccines unfortunately, the waning levels of antibodies comes with an ineffective immune response upon reexposure. As antibody levels following administration of the pertussis vaccine decline, it slowly becomes ineffective over the course of 10 years (Edwards, 2005). The solution to secondary vaccine failure is to administer booster doses when protection fades away. Research on COVID-19 has shown that in a majority of people who contracted the disease, developed antibodies diminished over the course of three months (Seow et al., 2020). On a more hopeful note, there is reason to believe that people may still retain immunity to COVID-19 for some time after developing antibodies through infection or vaccinations. There have been no cases where reinfection has explicitly happened. Although some cases of infection have been reported after recovery, it is believed that they are either due to false positives, or are lingering effects of the disease (Omer et al., 2020). Additionally, a reinfection study conducted in rhesus macaques confirmed that shortly after recovering from COVID-19, immunity is retained. After the monkeys recovered from the disease, reexposing them to SARS-CoV-2 did not cause infection, nor any COVID-19 symptoms (Bao et al., 2020). This is good news, as it demonstrates that a

COVID-19 vaccine can generate immunity, at least in the short term. However, as the disease is relatively new, it is still unknown whether an immune response generated through infection or vaccination can protect us in the long term. This is an aspect of the vaccine candidates that researchers will have to monitor over an extended period of time.

While there are many barriers to vaccine development, the efforts directed towards the eradication of COVID-19 are certainly progressing well. Clinical testing for several vaccines display signs of efficacy, lowering the chance of primary vaccine failures. Though antibody dependent enhancement may very well become an emergent issue with COVID-19, a number of vaccine candidates were able to induce working antibodies. Additionally, immunity to reinfection was proven for the short term. However, with all this optimism also comes a caveat. Only time can tell the long term effectiveness and safety of these vaccine candidates. It is plausible that immunity due to vaccination or previous infection could fade over time, possibly requiring improvements in the vaccines, or booster doses to maintain immunity. In regards to failure of vaccine effectiveness, vaccine technology is only half the story. The other half lies in the logistics of vaccine delivery. The absence of a solid system to deliver and administer vaccines would render even the best vaccines useless. Fortunately, there are logistical measures in development to distribute vaccines to the world.

Chapter 12 - Logistics of COVID-19 Vaccine Distribution

By: Jenny Gao

Post-Development and Distribution of the COVID-19 Vaccine

The end of the COVID-19 pandemic is reliant on finding a vaccine for the SARS-CoV-2 virus. However, development of the vaccine is only the beginning of a multifaceted operation to eradicate the spread of the disease. Take for example, the case of the mRNA-1273 vaccine candidate for the SARS-CoV-2 virus. On July 27th, 2020, biotechnology giant Moderna with the National Institute of Allergy and Infectious Diseases announced the distribution of 30 000 doses of its mRNA-1273 vaccine candidate. This distribution enters the vaccine into Phase III of clinical trials. In phase III of clinical trials, the vaccine will be distributed amongst 89 research sites across the United States. All sites involved are areas at high risk of infection by the SARS-CoV-2 virus. Moving towards the final stages of vaccine production before licensure, this clinical trial enrolls healthy volunteers through the database *ClinicalTrials.gov* in a randomized, placebo-controlled study (National Institutes of Health, 2020)

Including mRNA-1273, there are three vaccine candidates in phase III of clinical trials as of the start of August 2020. While the vaccine development process during the pandemic follows an accelerated time frame, post-vaccine production and distribution must also be accelerated. National agencies and governments will also have the difficult task to implement an effective vaccine distribution and accessibility plan during the COVID-19 pandemic. Hurdles in ending the COVID-19 pandemic could arise from stalls in distribution because of unavailable manufacturing facilities and a lack of funding in developing countries. Immunization for the SARS-CoV-2 virus will only be fully effective if enough people across the globe are vaccinated. Therefore, in this chapter we will explore the logistical struggles involved in global, equitable vaccine distribution. We will also explore the importance of global networks between private and publicly funded agencies to combat these barriers in vaccine distribution.

Tribulations in the Mass-Production of Vaccines

In previous chapters, we touched on the need for more manufacturing facilities to support the production of COVID-19 vaccines. An efficient network of private and public facilities for vaccine manufacturing is needed for global distribution for an accelerated time frame. Typically, manufacturing vaccines can take up to two years or even close to a decade when inefficient practices and inadequate techniques are practiced (Felter, 2020). The accelerated time frame during the COVID-19 pandemic calls for a manufacturing period of only three to six months. Therefore, it is in our best interest to analyze barriers in distributing mass doses of vaccines through both a modern and antiquated perspective. The licensure for an H1N1 vaccine was approved on October 5th, 2009, this was a positive stride towards the eradication of the H1N1 virus. During the H1N1 pandemic, the distribution of the H1N1 vaccine was halted by the tribulations that manufacturing companies experienced during production. At the end of January 2010, only 124 million doses of the H1N1 vaccine were available for global distribution during the pandemic. One of the problems with the mass production of the H1N1 vaccine was a lack of facilities available to complete the fill-finish steps of packaging the vaccines (Spiro & Emanuel, 2020). The fill-finish steps include filling of the vials with the vaccine product and the finished packaging of the product for distribution. From the beginning of the H1N1 vaccine production process, there was a lack of post-manufacturing facilities to accelerate the distribution of the vaccine. With the distribution delay, the H1N1 viral strain was able to mutate, and the public began to develop anti-vaccine sentiments. Similar problems with a lack of manufacturing facilities and therefore, the mutation of the COVID-19 virus can arise during this pandemic as well. These problems can cause delays in distribution by an additional few months, which may put thousands more lives at risk (McKenna, 2010). In order to avoid similar time delays and vaccine shortages like the H1N1 vaccine, there must be enough facilities running to meet the fill-finish steps during production of the COVID-19 vaccine.

Manufacturing Strategies and Investments

The aftermath of the H1N1 vaccine problem saw an investment of $400 million by the Biomedical Advanced Research and Development Authority (BARDA) of the United States in post-production resources. This investment worked to build partnerships between biotechnology firms, academic institutions and pharmaceutical companies in order to expand facilities for future mass vaccine production and research (McKenna, 2020). To prevent delays in the distribution of the COVID-19 vaccine, governments have also contracted pharmaceutical companies hundreds of millions to billions of dollars to use their facilities or to build new facilities to expedite the vaccine production process. In the United States, Operation Warp Speed was established by the Department of Health and Human Services (HHS) and the Department of Defense. This operation connects private manufacturers and industries with the federal agency to speed up the distribution of the COVID-19 vaccine. Private manufacturers such as Moderna, Pfizer, Johnson & Johnson, AstraZeneca and Novavax have all made contracts with the federal agency to accelerate and to accelerate the fill-finish orders during licensure. BARDA has also contracted with Emergent BioSolutions, a private manufacturing company, for the production of up to 1 billion doses of the COVID-19 vaccine by 2021 (this includes the fill-finish steps of production). In European countries such as the United Kingdom, university institutions including Oxford University have worked alongside government agencies to build the Vaccines Manufacturing and Innovations Center (VMIC UK). The VMIC UK is a scientific research company and manufacturing infrastructure committed to distributing COVID-19 vaccines by the summer of 2021 (Spiro & Emanuel, 2020).

Vaccine Platforms and Efficient Technology

In addition to expanding networks between public and private corporations for an accelerated vaccine distribution plan, the potential platforms for vaccine packaging and administration will play a role in the distribution timeframe and availability of the COVID-19 vaccine. If the vaccine can be administered in the single dose to achieve an effective immunity response, more people will be able to receive the vaccine. Immunity by a single dose schedule saves on both production and distribution. Platforms that elicit powerful immune responses in a single dose include live-attenuated vaccines as a candidate for the COVID-19 vaccine. However, these vaccines often cannot remain in high temperatures for long-term storage during distribution. Newer platforms such as viral vector vaccines have the potential to be single dose administrations as well, but some of these platforms still have the same problem with high temperatures and long-term storage (Spiro & Emanuel, 2020). To combat these temperature challenges, suitable materials such as glass vials and the freeze-drying technique can be used to prolong storage in remote areas without refrigeration (Spiro & Emanuel, 2020). Freeze-drying, also known as lyophilization, was used on the live-attenuated smallpox vaccines to prolong the effectiveness of the and microbial organisms in the product. Lyophilization refers to the fact that the freeze-drying technique works by removing water from the microbial organism or protein antigens in the vaccine. Simply put, the microbial organisms in the vaccine are placed in extremely low temperatures and frozen, then it is dried through a vacuuming process. In this process, the water is removed to transform the vaccine into a powder form which is more stable for long-term storage during its distribution (BioPharma, 2014). Another solution to maintain optimal conditions for vaccine potency (or cold chain storage) of single dose platforms includes the distribution of vaccines in glass vials. Manufacturing company Corning produces glass vials to hold vaccines during distribution;

the glass vials contain stabilizing chemicals in its packaging for cold chain storage. However, a major concern regarding glass vials is the amount that can be produced in an accelerated time frame. It is estimated that 660 million single dose vaccines would be needed for COVID-19 in the United States alone. Even after signing a contract with BARDA for its glass vial production, Corning would still only be able to administer 164 million vials per year. While other manufacturing companies including Johnson & Johnson have signed a contract with the Stevanato Group to produce another 250 million glass vials, this is still not enough for a worldwide distribution of the COVID-19 vaccine. To help push the distribution of the COVID-19 vaccine, researchers have been looking into alternative products and techniques to not only increase supply, but also to decrease the cost of production. One example of this is how the SiO2 Material Sciences company has received government funding to produce a cheaper vaccine vial and therefore increase supply. The company produces plastic vials with a layer of microscopic glass coating, so the packaging still maintains its cold chain system. However, the plastic vials are a relatively new technology compared to the glass vials, and its long-term effectiveness is still being researched. On the other hand, multidose vials are also being researched as a method to increase the quantity of vaccine doses produced and distributed as a result of less packaging required (Spiro & Emanuel, 2020). Johnson & Johnson have contracted Catalent Pharma Solutions in the United States to develop vials that are filled with ten doses of the vaccine instead of a single dose for faster production (Pagliusi et al., 2020). With enough funding, new techniques such as the use of patch application instead of needle applications with the COVID-19 vaccine could be used. Micro patch application is beneficial for distribution of vaccines in remote and low-income countries, as a medical clinician is not required for the administration of the vaccine (The College of Physicians of Philadelphia, 2018). In order to prevent delays in vaccine administration and to ensure that the maximum number of doses are distributed, both federal agencies and private manufacturers must research the most effective and cost-efficient materials and techniques to implement into their production processes.

Global Alliances for Vaccine Distribution

Inadequate accessibility and a lack of vaccine distribution to low income countries results in two million preventable deaths each year, two thirds of which are children under the age of five (Gowrisankar, 2020). In a global effort to eradicate the COVID-19 pandemic, nations around the globe must come together to ensure that vaccines are not stockpiled in developed countries and made unavailable to low and middle income countries. Yet, this challenge, as addressed by the Coalition for Epidemic Preparedness Innovations (CEPI) and the World Health Organization could require a global funding of $2 billion for manufacturing vaccine trials and an additional $1 billion for its global distribution (Khamsi, 2020). To assist with funding, the Developing Countries Vaccine Manufacturers Network (DCVMN) is a committee that joins 41 manufacturing members from developing countries to assist in manufacturing and distribution of the COVID-19 vaccine. Within the DCVMN, 13 members have been pre-qualified by the World Health Organization for meeting global distribution regulations. This could help accelerate the global distribution of the COVID-19 vaccine, especially with using pre-qualified members for approved practices in developing viral vector vaccines. The DCVMN has distributed vaccines to 170 developing countries and they are responsible for more than

65 percent of the vaccines produced outside of the American and European Regions approved by the World Health Organization (J. Rogers, 2020). Forming alliances between manufacturers in low-income countries, the DCVMN members are connected by the vaccine production process from research, manufacturing, supply, to administration. Important members of the committee that have developed COVID-19 vaccine candidates include Sinovac Biotech. This biopharmaceutical company does not have enough facilities for the mass manufacturing of its vaccine, but worked under DCVMN to outsource their technology to other members. In order to accelerate global distribution, members of DCVMN are committed to reserving 50 percent of their existing capacity for manufacturing COVID-19 vaccines after accounting for stockpiles of various other vaccines. On June 22nd, 2020, the DCVMN reported that 14 of their members have spare capacities for the immediate manufacturing including vaccine formulation, labelling, packaging, storage and distribution (Pagliusi et al., 2020).

Additionally, the World Health Organization, CEPI and GAVI have established a COVID-19 vaccine global access facility known as COVAX as part of their R&D blueprint effort. COVAX will incorporate networks between large pharmaceutical companies, private donors and public financial sectors of developed countries to contribute to the distribution of a guaranteed share of doses for all countries. The goal of COVAX will be to distribute 950 million doses of the COVID-19 vaccine to low-income countries and 950 million doses to high-income countries. In order to meet their goal, COVAX has encouraged contracts between large pharmaceutical companies with manufacturing facilities in developing countries (Gavi, n.d.).

The benefits for these companies to push research and facilities in developing countries include a reduction in cost for labor and production as well as raw materials (Chokshi et al., 2020).

Distribution Techniques

Administration strategies from healthcare providers and the tracking of doses must be improved to increase the amount of people vaccinated for COVID-19. After a COVID-19 vaccine gets approved by the National Advisory Committee on Immunization (NACI), Canadians will be able to receive doses through their healthcare providers. In the United States, the COVID-19 vaccine will be approved by the Food and Drug Administration (FDA) before doses are made available to the public and private healthcare providers. The struggle of vaccine distribution then arises from a lack of government funding for public clinics and clinician hours available to administer doses. For instance, in the United States, private providers have been referring patients to public healthcare sectors for vaccine administrations. However, there is limited state funding for local healthcare providers to purchase adequate amounts of vaccine doses. Additionally, there are limited numbers of public providers in some states. For example, Oklahoma only had five federally qualified health care centers running 18 sites in its state. In the United States, around 27.9 million citizens are uninsured and therefore can only receive the COVID-19 vaccine through a public healthcare site. In clinics, it takes around 3.5 minutes for a health professional to administer a single dose vaccine. To put into perspective, it would take a total of 3.2 million hours each year to administer vaccines for just a cohort of children in the United States. Public healthcare sites must receive more vaccine doses and support for clinicians during COVID-19 vaccine distribution because of the spillover of patients from private sectors. The Advisory Committee on Immunization Practices should consider expanding budgeting on more vaccine doses for public clinics and pediatrician offices to more quickly administer COVID-19 vaccines. (Institute of Medicine, 2003).

An accelerated model for vaccine production processes can shorten the manufacturing and distribution timeframe of doses from the normal 3 years to a mere 7 months (Felter, 2020). With 18 million positive cases of SARS-CoV-2 virus and 700 000 related deaths confirmed globally as of August 2020, global accessibility and the acceleration of vaccine administration will save thousands of lives (Pagliusi et al., 2020). In developed countries such as the United States, 660 million single doses of the COVID-19 vaccine is required for distribution according to BARDA. Yet, the challenge of maintaining herd immunity in global networks requires equity for every country during vaccine distribution for COVID-19. Partnerships between CEPI, GAVI, the Gates Foundation and large pharmaceutical companies bring action to the goal for 2 billion doses of COVID-19 vaccine to be distributed by the end of 2021 (Spiro & Emanuel, 2020). Therefore, both international organizations and government sectors of countries must focus research and funding on post-development techniques and initiatives for COVID-19 vaccine distribution.

Chapter 13 - Ethics of Distribution

By: Ivy Quan

The development of a safe and efficacious vaccine is only half the battle, and efforts will be futile without being able to scale up production and ensure equitable distribution. In the previous chapter, we discussed major logistical challenges associated with vaccine production and distribution, and how those challenges almost guarantee vaccine shortages at least in the preliminary stages of distribution. When these shortages occur, we will inevitably see how underlying geopolitical and socioeconomic forces affect vaccine distribution both internationally and nationally. On the international stage, it's easy to see how a majority of the vaccine supply could be held by the world's wealthiest countries. The ever increasing demand may ultimately lead to an increase in prices, so the wealthiest countries will be able to procure the most doses, leaving little left for developing countries. Who is responsible for ensuring that the needs of developing countries are also met? Even within a country, equitable distribution of a vaccine is difficult. Who should get vaccinated first, and how will the governments of each country determine priority? In this chapter, we will discuss the moral and ethical challenges of vaccine distribution alongside some potential solutions. Though this may generate more questions than answers, lawmakers and public health officials must consider these ethical questions to ensure equitable distribution of a COVID-19 vaccine.

International Struggles

Anticipated shortages of a COVID-19 vaccine is a concern for world leaders who have been scrambling to secure vaccine supplies for their citizens ever since clinical trials began showing promising results. Many vaccine manufacturers have already signed contracts with countries such as the United States and the United Kingdom. Pfizer, in partnership with BioNTech and Fosun Pharma, signed a 1.95 billion-dollar contract with the U.S. to provide 100 million doses of their RNA vaccine, with the option to purchase an additional 500 million doses down the line (Erman & Banerjee, 2020). Pfizer and BioNTech have also agreed to provide the U.K. with 30 million vaccine doses at an undisclosed price (Erman & Banerjee 2020). AstraZeneca, in partnership with Oxford University, agreed to provide Britain with 100 million doses, giving Britain first access to their developing adenovirus vector vaccine. AstraZeneca also plans to receive 1.2 billion dollars from the U.S. government for 300 million doses ("AstraZeneca takes," 2020). While these are just a couple of examples, the common theme amongst these contracts and agreements is that wealthy countries who can afford to invest in development and manufacturing are bidding for early vaccine access. Although the rapid development and testing of COVID-19 vaccine candidates would not be possible without immense public and private financial backing from developed nations, this creates a dynamic where wealthy countries are prioritized and the needs of developing countries are easily forgotten. In an attempt to outbid each other for a vaccine, wealthy countries may also drive prices up, which would further impede equitable distribution.

What we are seeing here is coined vaccine nationalism. Countries take a "me first" approach and consider their own citizens as their sole obligation. While it is understandable that country leaders would want to take care of their residents first, this lack of international coordination is detrimental to any plans of global equitable vaccine distribution. We can compare this to the rule with oxygen masks on a flight - put yours on before assisting others. However, the problem arises when the entire supply of masks only drop down in the first class cabin and those with wealth and power get to choose when and how to distribute them to everyone else. This struggle has already played out with the drug Remdesivir.

Remdesivir, an antiviral medication from the company Gilead, is the only drug therapy approved to provide relief for those with severe COVID-19 symptoms thus far. As soon as it was approved for emergency use by the FDA, the U.S. bought 500,000 doses - almost Gilead's entire stock of the drug for three months (Boseley, 2020b). In response, Gilead signed a contract with Pfizer to help manufacture remdesivir to meet global demand (Loveface, 2020).
 Had Gilead not signed a deal with Pfizer, virtually no other country would have access to it, or at the very least, would have the drug in short supply until Gilead finishes producing the 500,000 doses for the U.S. in October of 2020. This "America first" mindset and their seeming unwillingness to cooperate with other countries hint at major challenges of equitable vaccine distribution. This attitude, seen amongst some high-income

countries, prioritises low-risk individuals in developed nations over high-risk populations in developing nations, which may prolong the pandemic.

In addition to vaccine nationalism, profit-driven vaccine companies also contribute to the challenges of vaccine distribution. Part of the reason why wealthier countries have disproportionate access to vaccines is because the vaccines' expensive prices are controlled by the vaccine companies. Although AstraZeneca and Johnson & Johnson both promised not to sell their vaccines at a profit for the first phase of the pandemic, Pfizer/BioNTech, Moderna, and Merck all expressed intentions on profiting from their vaccines. Moderna's president, Stephen Hoge, explicitly stated that Moderna "will not sell it at cost" (Wu, 2020). These different attitudes can be seen in the approximate costs for vaccine doses: Pfizer/BioNTech's RNA vaccine will cost roughly $19.5 per dose, and Moderna's RNA vaccine will cost around $25-$30 per dose, while AstraZeneca/Oxford University's adenovirus vector vaccine will cost a mere $4 per dose (Mancini, Cookson, & Kuchler, 2020). We discuss these companies in particular because they are all participating in Operation Warp Speed - a program by the U.S. government that provides promising vaccine candidates access to federal funds.

This inevitably raises some ethical questions: do companies that accept taxpayer funding have an obligation to make their vaccines as affordable as possible? In the U.S., Democratic lawmakers suggested that vaccine companies receiving federal funds should follow AstraZeneca and Johnson & Johnson to provide their vaccines not-for-profit ("Letter from James E. Clyburn," 2020). They were worried that Pfizer had not accepted any federal funds because it could lead to price gouging. The Daraprim price hike controversy is an extreme example of a pharmaceutical company's ability to gouge prices. In 2015, Martin Shkreli, founder of Turing Pharmaceuticals, acquired the drug Daraprim from Impax Laboratories. As part of the agreement, Impax withdrew the drug from pharmacies and adopted a strict, tightly controlled distribution. This effectively limited the supply of Daraprim. Once Turing took over the drug, Shkreli leveraged the limited supply to increase the price from $13.50 to $750 per pill (Pollack, 2015). At the time, there were no manufacturers making generic versions of Daraprim, and with limited competition, patients and insurance companies were forced to pay the price. This controversy shows how companies can take advantage of limited supplies to unethically generate immense profit. With limited supplies and global demand for a COVID-19 vaccine, it is easy to see how manufacturers can hike up prices for their own profit. This is why Democratic lawmakers in the U.S., in discussion with the Pharmaceutical Research Manufacturers of America (PhRMA), requested that "no drug company should be allowed to profiteer, especially during this public health emergency" ("Letter from James E. Clyburn," 2020). However, neither PhRMA nor its member companies provided any assurance of such plans. The decision of some companies to maintain high profit margins through a global pandemic may be seen as unethical by some people because it limits vaccine access to nations who can afford it.

International Organizations

In order to overcome this pandemic, vaccines need to be allocated to areas with the highest risk of infection. Unfortunately, most of the countries disproportionately affected by COVID-19 are low or middle-income nations. If these countries lag behind in procuring vaccine supplies, the risk of global transmission will persist and the virus will continue to impede global economies. Therefore, it is in everyone's best interest to collaborate and equitably distribute vaccines to reduce risk of infection around the world. The World Health Organization (WHO) has launched a massive, unprecedented global collaboration effort called The Access to COVID-19 Tools Accelerator (ACT-Accelerator). ACT-Accelerator joins the forces of governments, researchers, and philanthropists across the world to expedite the development, manufacturing, and fair distribution of testing kits, therapeutics and vaccines. The initiative consists of four pillars: diagnostics, treatments, vaccines, and health care system strengthening ("The Access," n.d.). The vaccine pillar aims to acquire and distribute 2 billion doses to low income countries. Leading the vaccine pillar of the ACT-Accelerator are two international organizations: The Coalition for Epidemic Preparedness Innovations (CEPI) and Gavi, The Vaccine Alliance (referred to as GAVI). Both are implementing frameworks to increase vaccine accessibility in low and middle income countries; CEPI through funding, and GAVI through distribution.

CEPI is an organization founded after the Ebola epidemic to assist the world in preparing for future global health emergencies. During COVID-19, they have attempted to ensure fair access to the vaccines while funding and accelerating vaccine development. CEPI uses donations from public and private sectors to fund the development and production of vaccines; however, they commit to equitable access by enforcing several policies upon companies receiving CEPI funding. These policies include: having a transparent methodology to determine vaccine price, committing to producing affordable products, allocating vaccines in a way that prioritizes populations that need it most, and overall, committing to equitable access (Huneycutt et al., 2020). By implementing these policies, CEPI can ethically fund vaccine companies and influence fair vaccine allocation and equitable access.

GAVI is a twenty-year-old organization that provides immunization programmes for those living in impoverished countries, particularly children. As part of the WHO's ACT-Accelerator program, GAVI has developed the COVID-19 Global Vaccine Access Facility (COVAX Facility) - a risk management tool that encourages global collaboration (Berkley, 2020). The COVAX Facility essentially acts as an insurance policy for manufacturers. All participating countries can pool their buying power to provide incentive for vaccine companies to scale up manufacturing. Scaling manufacturing during clinical trials is unprecedented and risky because the efficacy and safety of the vaccine candidate is still unknown. However, having countries across the world pool funding commitments ensures that there is sufficient demand, mitigating some of the inherent risks for vaccine manufacturers. On the other hand, scaling manufacturing will increase the number of doses available once a vaccine is licensed, which provides a base for equitable access. Global collaboration also tempers vaccine nationalism and promotes fair allocation of resources internationally. To assist lower income nations, GAVI launched the Gavi Advance Market Commitment for COVID-19 Vaccines (Gavi COVAX AMC) at the 2020 Global Vaccine Summit. Gavi COVAX AMC strives for affordable vaccines and global immunization by inviting donors to pool resources to procure and deliver vaccines for developing nations. As of July 2020, 75 developed countries expressed interest in funding 90 developing countries that qualify for funding, and GAVI has collected $500 million to purchase and deliver vaccines ("Gavi announces," 2020). AstraZeneca was the first company to sign an agreement with Gavi COVAX AMC and agreed to supply 300 million doses to countries funded by GAVI ("Gavi launches," 2020). This cements AstraZeneca and Oxford University's commitment to a globally accessible COVID-19 vaccine. Through the COVAX Facility and COVAX AMC, GAVI may mitigate some of the ethical issues surrounding vaccine distribution by encouraging global cooperation, increasing manufacturing of doses, and funding the procurement and distribution of vaccines to low income countries.

National Struggles

Equitable distribution is not only imperative across the world, but also within each country. Different communities and populations have varying levels of risks associated with COVID-19, which needs to be taken into account when allocating scarce vaccine resources. To get a sense of how governments have responded to vaccine shortages in the past, we can take a look at the United States' response during the H1N1 Influenza pandemic in 2009. The CDC Advisory Committee on Immunization Practices (ACIP) created priority groups to receive the vaccine first if supply was limited. Amongst the top priority were health care and emergency medical services personnel. This makes sense because health care workers, especially those on the frontlines, form the foundation of a nation's health care system and are integral in administering the vaccine. They are also at higher risk of exposure to the virus, so a top priority designation is well founded. Along with medical personnel, other priority groups included: pregnant women, those in contact with children under

6 months of age, children 6 months-4 years of age, and children 5-18 years of age with chronic medical conditions (Centers for Disease Control and Prevention, 2009). Although the priority groups will be different for the COVID-19 vaccine, we can investigate the reasoning behind these priority groups as a guide for the COVID-19 priority groups. While the H1N1 response prioritized those at high risk of infection and those at high risk of developing complications, the COVID-19 response may prioritize frontline healthcare workers, essential workers, seniors, and people with comorbid medical conditions such as cardiovascular disease, diabetes, or cancer ("People who are at high risk," 2020).

Another consideration for COVID-19 would be prioritizing vaccination in lower-income communities experiencing higher rates of infection and death. Often, these communities include people of colour who have been economically devastated by the pandemic. This is an important consideration because COVID-19 has resulted in mass unemployment and has put economies at a standstill. Unfair distribution of vaccines across socioeconomic lines can widen economic disparities within communities; once companies begin to rehire, an individual's status of immunization may be an important factor they consider. Since our return to normalcy is dependent on a safe and effective vaccine, the distribution of vaccines within countries must be carefully considered. Therefore, in creating priority groups to receive a vaccine, governments must not only consider the risk of infection or the risk of medical complications, but also the economic impact of COVID-19.

All in all, the development and production of vaccines is fruitless if those vaccines are not distributed ethically and equitably across the world. However grim it may be, we know one thing for sure: when vaccines first become available the supply will be dwarfed by the demand. When that occurs, countries can either bid each other out in a display of vaccine nationalism, or they can collaborate with the frameworks provided by the WHO, CEPI, GAV. If countries engage in vaccine nationalism, the winners of the bids are predictable, and the needs of the low income countries will be readily forgotten. We are not safe until everyone is; global health emergencies require global collaboration. Within countries, we should prioritize not only those who are medically at risk, but also those hit hardest economically. The bottom line is that we need world leaders to collaborate with each other and vaccine companies to prioritize people's health and safety over profit.

Chapter 14 - Vaccine Hesitancy and COVID-19

By: Evangelea Touliopoulos

While it is true that in order for a COVID-19 vaccine to be effective, it needs to be distributed to everyone regardless of what country they are from and how much money or power they possess, one thing that cannot be ignored is that even if everyone were to have access to a COVID-19 vaccine tomorrow, there would still be a multitude of people who would choose not to get vaccinated for a variety of reasons. This could put the effectiveness of the vaccine in jeopardy and allow for future small outbreaks of the virus in areas with low vaccination rates. It also brings up many ethical debates about vaccination in general, such as how far the government should go to encourage people to get vaccinated.

Religious Reasons People Choose Not to Get Vaccinated

Understanding the variety of reasons that people refuse vaccination is important so that high risk groups can be identified and innovative solutions could potentially be found that could encourage vaccination in these groups. The most common reason that vaccination is refused is cited as religious reasons (McKee & Bohannon, 2016). Typically, people with religious beliefs against getting vaccinated usually refuse all vaccines for themselves and their children, so it is unlikely that they will choose to use a COVID-19 vaccine (McKee & Bohannon, 2016). However, there are several different reasons that a variety of religions refuse vaccination, so some of these reasons may apply to the COVID-19 vaccine and others may not.

In Catholicism, there is a moral objection to vaccines that use cell lines derived from voluntarily aborted fetuses (Pelčić et al., 2016). This is because abortion is considered a sin by many devout Catholics, making them against the use of any product made using anything derived from voluntarily aborted fetuses (Pelčić et al., 2016). Some examples of common vaccines that use these cell lines are the vaccines for rubella, chickenpox, smallpox, and hepatitis (Pelčić et al., 2016). However, Catholicism does not have a completely black and white view on the subject. Since many Catholics recognize that these vaccines save lives, many believe that it is morally right to take them to protect themselves and others. However, there still exists a subset of Catholics who refuse to use vaccines with any connection to voluntary abortion. Considering that several of the lead candidates for a COVID-19 vaccine use cell lines derived from aborted fetuses, such as Oxford's AZD1222, Moderna's mRNA-1273, and Johnson & Johnson's Ad26.COV2-S, there is the possibility that a subset of Catholics may refuse them (Abbamonte, 2020). However, there is also the possibility that a COVID-19 vaccine will be created without using cell lines that were derived from an aborted fetus, which means that people of the Catholic faith should have no problem using them. Some potential COVID-19 vaccine candidates that do not use these controversial cell lines are developed by Novavax and Sinovac (Abbamonte, 2020).

Another religion with potential objections to vaccines is Protestantism (Ruijs et al., 2012). Some people of Protestant faith refuse vaccines because they believe that vaccines are inappropriate as they interfere with God's will (Ruijs et al., 2012). Many think that God should be the one to decide if their children and themselves should be spared from a virus (Ruijs et al., 2012). There are also accounts of people who recount being thankful for their experience with infection because they claim that it brought them closer to God (Ruijs et al., 2012). People with this belief will often be willing to accept curative measures, but not preventative ones (such as vaccines). This means they could potentially be willing to accept a vaccine during a pandemic because it could be seen as curative since the threat of the virus is already on them instead of it being something that could happen sometime in the future (Ruijs et al., 2012). However, there is still the possibility that some members of this community could refuse a potential COVID-19 vaccine.

Those of Buddhist faith may also have objections to vaccination (Pelčić et al., 2016). In Buddhism, it is believed that all life and all life forms are related to each other and it is therefore believed that one should never intentionally kill any living creature (Pelčić et al., 2016).
This could be problematic with respect to vaccines, as vaccines can often be derived from animal products, which means that Buddhists may oppose them (Pelčić et al., 2016). However, most

modern Buddhists will use vaccines anyways, as they see them as a way to ensure that their health and the health of those around them is protected (Pelčić et al., 2016).

One important thing to remember with respect to religion and vaccine hesitancy is that none of these religions have outright opposed vaccines. Instead, it is individual members who are applying their own religious beliefs to vaccination and drawing their own conclusions. It is also crucial to note that the majority of people who practice the religions mentioned in this chapter do choose to vaccinate themselves and their families, but it is still important to understand the reasoning behind those who interpret their religion in a way that opposes vaccination.

Other Reasons to Refuse Vaccination

Concerns around safety is another primary reason why parents may choose not to vaccinate their children. Over the past few years, there has been a growing movement that believes that vaccines are dangerous. With the help of the internet, there has been a lot of misinformation about vaccines being circulated to parents, as well as genuine risks that have been exaggerated and sensationalized. For example, a popular belief among those who are worried about vaccination is that vaccines can cause autism (DeStefano & Shimabukuro, 2019). The vaccine that is implicated in this controversy is the Measles, Mumps, and Rubella (MMR) vaccine (DeStefano & Shimabukuro, 2019). There was a since retracted study published in 1998 that linked the MMR vaccine to autism (DeStefano & Shimabukuro, 2019). This study prompted a variety of inquiries into the relationship between the MMR vaccine and autism, all of which found that the MMR vaccine does not increase the prevalence of autism (DeStefano &

Shimabukuro, 2019). However, this original study received plenty of media coverage which caused a significant amount of the public to lose confidence in vaccines (DeStefano & Shimabukuro, 2019). In the United Kingdom, shortly after the controversial study was published, MMR vaccination rates dropped from around 90% to 80% (DeStefano & Shimabukuro, 2019). As a result, the number of measles cases in the U.K. increased twenty-fold (DeStefano & Shimabukuro, 2019). This shows how dangerous misinformation about vaccines can be. This hesitancy over the MMR vaccine has been generalized to other vaccines. Several people believe that vaccines can lead to many different health complications, such as brain damage, behavioral problems, and other severe adverse reactions (McKee & Bohannon, 2016). The media can often worsen these fears by reporting on the rare adverse reactions that do occur with vaccination, which feeds into the public's fear. Furthermore, in developed countries, many of the pathogens that we vaccinate against are almost completely eradicated, so people forget how dangerous they were before the development of vaccines. Many parents believe that even if their child contracts the pathogen, they will fight it off naturally like they would fight a common cold (McKee & Bohannon, 2016). Unfortunately, this selfish line of thinking could prove to be disastrous. Outbreaks of previously eradicated diseases in developed countries, such as smallpox, have been increasing in recent years (DeStefano & Shimabukuro, 2019).

However, since the threat of the SARS-CoV-2 virus is much more prominent than a lot of the other pathogens that vaccines work against, there is a possibility that there will be less vaccine hesitancy due to safety concerns. Since people are more likely to be seeing the detrimental effects of the virus, they may be more likely to decide that the vaccine is worth the risk. Unfortunately, there will always be people who will decide not to vaccinate for a variety of safety concerns, but that number will hopefully be minimal for the COVID-19 vaccine.

COVID-19 and the Harmful Effects of Vaccine Hesitancy

In order for the COVID-19 pandemic to be controlled, there needs to be a high percentage of the population that is vaccinated. If many people chose not to get vaccinated, and especially if those people live clustered together, outbreaks of the virus will continue, prolonging the pandemic. This could be very dangerous to people who medically cannot get vaccinated due to compromised immune systems or severe reactions to vaccines, such as allergies to vaccine components. In order for a vaccine to be maximally effective in a community, herd immunity must be fulfilled. Herd immunity occurs when enough members of a community become immune to a specific pathogen, minimizing the spread from person to person (Mayo Clinic, n.d.). This allows the whole community to be protected. The percentage of people that need to be immune to the disease for herd immunity to work changes depending on how contagious the pathogen is (Mayo Clinic, n.d.). For COVID-19, it is estimated that 70-90% of the population would need to be vaccinated in order to successfully have herd immunity, depending on the efficacy of the vaccine (L. Rogers & Health, n.d.). However, one thing to consider is that since many people who choose not to get vaccinated live in communities with others who share the same beliefs as them, it is possible that there will be outbreaks of the SARS-CoV-2 virus in those communities because of the low vaccination rates. This is similar to the way there was a measles outbreak in the Jewish Orthodox community in New York City in 2018 and 2019 (Zucker et al., 2020). Many in the Jewish Orthodox community chose not to vaccinate, so when one child brought home measles from Israel, it spread rapidly and 649 cases of measles were confirmed in the following 10 months (Zucker et al., 2020). If communities exist with low vaccination rates for COVID-19, similar outbreaks will most likely continue to occur in those communities for years. The outbreaks can also affect people who do not live in the community, but who are medically unable to get vaccinated, as they may get infected when interacting with unvaccinated people in public.

Ethical Concerns About Vaccination Regulations

These concerns about herd immunity bring up the question of whether the government should create regulations with regards to COVID-19 vaccination for the medically sound. This can be done by only allowing access to school, work, or public locations to vaccinated individuals. There already exists a list of vaccines that children must receive to be able to attend school, but children are allowed to be excluded from vaccination if they claim religious reasons. There is much debate on how strict the regulations for vaccination should be to ensure everyone's safety without infringing on societal freedoms. For instance, in Ontario, to be exempt from vaccination people must visit a local public health unit and complete an education session that covers vaccine safety and the risks of not getting vaccinated (Ontario, 2015). In the United States, it varies state by state, but people are usually able to claim religious reasons without much effort (Pelčić et al., 2016). Considering the immediate danger that the SARS-CoV-2 virus poses, should there be stricter guidelines for getting exemptions from the vaccine? Another thing to consider is that all adults need to be vaccinated as well. There are not very many regulations on vaccination for adults, unless you work in healthcare or with other vulnerable populations. This virus brings up the question of whether some regulations should be implemented to ensure that enough members of our communities are vaccinated to achieve herd immunity. However, enforcing stricter regulations is sure to cause outcry among members of our communities who are opposed to vaccines, so the challenge is to find the correct balance.

Even though vaccines have made an enormous positive impact on the health of our communities and have eliminated many previously dangerous threats, they are still considered a fairly controversial topic. It is important to understand why people may oppose vaccines in order to create regulations and initiatives that will increase vaccination rates and will thus make our communities healthier and safer. This is especially true during the COVID-19 pandemic as we can see the devastating effects that occur when communities lack immunity for a dangerous pathogen. However, the SARS-CoV-2 virus can be used as a teaching moment that demonstrates what happens when vaccines do not exist for viruses. This may help people realize the necessity of vaccination. Furthermore, the positive effects of a SARS-CoV-2 vaccine will be blatantly obvious, which may also help to encourage people to get vaccinated. Hopefully, when a vaccine for COVID-19 is readily available, enough people will get vaccinated to achieve herd immunity, and subsequently, trust in vaccines may improve, improving public health for years to come.

Chapter 15 - World Health Relations and Vaccine Diplomacy

By: Jenny Gao

International health policies and cooperation between governing nations became a legitimized effort on July 23rd, 1851. The first International Sanitary Conference in Paris, France was held on that date and paved the way for the succession of 13 conferences to follow. During these meetings, administrators and scientists exchanged medical and health diplomacy ideas (World Health Organization, 2011). It was through this conference that the idea of vaccine diplomacy and vaccine science diplomacy would originate (Hotez, 2014). These two important terms will be defined in the paragraphs to follow. The history involved in building world health relations and establishing vaccine diplomacy will highlight strategies and operations that can be conducted by countries during the COVID-19 pandemic. This chapter will touch on the efforts put forth in formulating world relations during the COVID-19 pandemic that will impact the global production process of the COVID-19 vaccine. We will also explore world relation efforts to help developing and war-torn countries that are at high risk during the COVID-19 pandemic. In an effort to determine the most effective strategy for global vaccine administration and its diplomacy, we will also explore the trade relations between countries during the COVID-19 pandemic.

The History of Health Diplomacy

As philosopher George Santayana states, "Those who cannot remember the past are condemned to repeat it." (Magritte, 1905).

Evidently, we must first understand how international health cooperation was formed and the reasons behind its formation in order to understand how COVID-19 vaccine diplomacy may be carried out. Simply put, vaccine diplomacy refers to the international health policies and relationships that are involved in the production, distribution, and usage of vaccines. This form of diplomacy has another subsection known as vaccine science diplomacy. Vaccine science diplomacy includes the ideas and efforts between medical professionals and scientists with administrators to develop and share technologies and suggestions during the production, distribution and usage of vaccines (Hotez, 2014). Both forms of diplomacy have been exercised during the accelerated efforts of the COVID-19 vaccine production process.

Disease control and infection prevention efforts can be traced back to the 14th century in the Adriatic Coasts of Croatia (Hotez, 2014). Dr. Edward Jenner demonstrated vaccine science diplomacy when he administered his cowpox vaccine to treat smallpox in patients after being granted permission from governments in Russia, Spain, Turkey and Native American tribes in Canada, the United States and Mexico (Hotez, 2014).

This was an early display of vaccine science diplomacy as Jenner shared his smallpox vaccine platform internationally. Towards the end of the 19th century, scientist Louis Pasteur reasoned that science is universal and belongs to everyone, especially in the form of healthcare. He established the Pasteur Institute in France and worked to create laboratories in Francophone countries in Indochina and North Africa to distribute the rabies vaccine universally. From 1892 to 1897, a scientist by the name of Dr. Waldemar Haffkine travelled to India in order to distribute his cholera and plague vaccine and he established the Haffkine Institute in Mumbai to continue scientific research (Hotez, 2014). In the same century, the first International Sanitary Conference was held between European nations to address the cholera epidemic. At the conference, countries and diplomats joined together in order to develop a safe and cost-efficient plan to implement maritime quarantine across the European nations. The plague pandemic was also discussed in 1897 at the tenth International Sanitary Conference in an effort to contain the outbreak. Further world relations and international health policies were formed in 1907 when the permanent health bureau, Office international d'Hygiène publique (OIHP), was formed by health and government officials (World Health Organization, 2011).

Shortly after World War I, the League of Nations was created in a global diplomacy effort and also focused on disease prevention and control, working alongside OIHP. Most international health diplomacy efforts were placed on hold during World War II and resumed after the United Nations was formed when nations met in San Francisco and made suggestions for international health policies. After writing these propositions, the Constitution of the World Health Organization (WHO) was signed on July 22nd, 1946 by 51 members of the United Nations (World Health Organization, 2011). The WHO has since taken on worldwide eradication campaigns and is the leading agency for international public health. The WHO has been the spearhead in the R&D efforts (research and development) and international collaboration on all information relating to COVID-19 and COVID-19 immunization (World Health Organization, 2020).

Throughout history, tensions between nations caused strains on world health relations. Yet, vaccine science diplomacy was still practiced and saved the lives of millions of people during these periods of hardship. For instance, the Cold War between the United States and the Union of Soviet Socialists Republic (USSR) caused geopolitical tensions. However, from 1956 to 1959, Dr. Albert Sabin from the United States worked together with Dr. Mikhail Chumakov from the USSR to develop the oral polio vaccine. They reasoned with diplomats and government officials between the two strained nations to allow the administration of their polio vaccine to 10 million children in the USSR, and then to 100 million adolescents. This oral polio vaccine was crucial to the eradication campaign for the outbreak of the polio virus. After the Cold War, the continuation of vaccine science diplomacy was practiced by the nations involved in developing the freeze-dried vaccine, an important technique for vaccine storage. From 1962 to 1966, the USSR developed the lyophilization technique to store live-attenuated smallpox vaccines for long periods of time. Working with the eradication campaign directed by the WHO, the USSR developed this method with funding from the United States (Hotez, 2014).

Multidimensions in COVID-19 Vaccine Diplomacy

Entering the 21st century, vaccine diplomacy and world health relations expanded with the continued work of the WHO, the United Nations, and other global agencies. Such actions will be helpful in the global effort to end the COVID-19 pandemic. There are three general categories used to classify global health diplomacy (Hotez, 2014). The first category includes the core diplomacy of nations and governments that are involved in classic Westphalian systems of negotiating and building policies. The second category involved in world health relations includes agencies that network and cooperate between nations; these are international agencies that include the WHO, the Gavi Alliance and other non-government organizations (NGOs). Informal members of diplomacy are involved in the third category of global health relations; these can be scientific partnerships and private funders including the Bill & Melinda Gates Foundation (Hotez, 2014). It is important to recognize the multidimensionality involved with world health relations as it will prove to be useful in the R&D Blueprint efforts for COVID-19 immunization.

Several large-industrial holding countries have threatened the multilateral efforts that the WHO and other international agencies have implemented to end the COVID-19 pandemic. For instance, critics have accused the World Health Organization of being too privy in their delayed announcement of the COVID-19 virus as a public health emergency and a pandemic. Furthermore, the President of the United States, Donald Trump, criticized China's involvement in the outbreak of the COVID-19 pandemic as the virus originated from Wuhan, China. As tension between the United States and China grew since the COVID-19 outbreak, Trump has criticized the WHO in their influence from China.

As a result, on May 29th, 2020, the United States announced its withdrawal of funding for the WHO and its potentially permanent leave as a member of the international organization. The United States has provided the WHO $450 million in annual funding for its immunization work. Efforts to accelerate the production of the COVID-19 vaccine and the global distribution of its doses will be negatively affected by this decision (Nature. Editorial, 2020). The WHO, alongside other agencies of vaccine diplomacy, are responsible for large scale vaccine campaigns and remain operating through governmental funding – the United States being a major financier for these organizations. With estimates of economic growth to drop by 3-6% and global trade to decline by 13-32% in 2020, funding for the WHO may further decrease. As the Lancet reports, only population-wide immunity against the COVID-19 virus may lead to the economic restoration and the return of daily life around the world. Therefore, the health of the global nation is reliant on a vaccine program overseen by the WHO (Gellin, 2020). In response to the United States' withdrawal of funding, China has donated $2 billion to the WHO and has promised medical supplies to developing countries during the pandemic. Additionally, U.S. Congress has confirmed any contributions and funding already contracted to the WHO cannot be taken back within a year's notice of the United States' retraction. While the United States' government may wish to withdraw from the WHO, there is an option for the United States to resume its support for the organization in the future. Referencing back to the Cold War, in 1949, the USSR was not impressed with the dominance that the United States had as a member of the WHO, and wanted to permanently leave their position on the committee. It was Canadian Brock Chisholm, director-general of the WHO at that time, that suggested the

USSR be "inactivated" instead of permanently withdrawn from the committee so that they can return in future years. Similar measures can be implemented again in 2020 should the United States wish to leave the organization but return to support health initiatives in the future (Nature. Editorial, 2020).

COVID-19 Calls for a Ceasefire

Humanitarian efforts made as a part of world health relations are also important during the COVID-19 pandemic, especially with respect to the distribution of vaccines. The efforts involved in vaccine diplomacy include actions of ceasefire in developing and war-torn countries during vaccination campaigns. The WHO and the United Nations Children's Fund (UNICEF) work to resolve hostile situations in war-torn countries with great efforts to vaccinate children (Hotez, 2014). Henrietta Fore, UNICEF's executive director in 2020, urged countries currently at war to call a ceasefire so that children of those countries will be able to receive the COVID-19 vaccine when it is distributed. The ceasefire would mean that the children in war-torn countries would be protected from being killed, maimed, or removed from their homes. The ceasefire also spares healthcare infrastructures and open-neutral spaces from being destroyed to allow essential healthcare workers to administer the COVID-19 vaccine safely (United Nations, 2020). This call-to-action can be implemented through the Humanitarian Cease-Fire Project (HCFP), which mediates in war-torn countries to offer immunization and food supplies to civilians. The HCFP has negotiated for Days of Tranquility, which has allowed provisions and nutritional packages to enter the war-torn countries. As well, through the Sanctuaries for Peace, medical and health care infrastructures in those countries will be protected for the distribution of vaccines.

For instance, from March 13th to 19th, 2001, the HCFP was able to negotiate a deal between the Taliban and the Northern Alliance to allow UNICEF and the WHO to administer their immunization campaign to civilians (World Health Organization, 2012). When observing world health relations and responses, it is clear that humanitarian efforts made by international organizations is an important component to global immunization for the COVID-19 pandemic. As a result of these humanitarian efforts during the COVID-19 pandemic, eleven war-torn countries have agreed to temporary ceasefires. This agreement will save hundreds of thousands of children from death caused by the COVID-19 in countries such as Afghanistan, Burkina Faso, Libya, Mali, Myanmar, Syria, Ukraine and Yemen (United Nations, 2020).

Countries around the world have stretched their resources and vaccine industries in response to the COVID-19 pandemic. Monopoly agreements between large pharmaceutical industries and manufacturers of different countries have been made, and nations have shown interest in the equitable distribution of vaccine doses to low and middle-income countries. Yet each country will look after their own citizens and political interests first. For instance, in April 2020, the United States restricted N95 respiratory mask exports to Canada in order to keep medical supplies for themselves. Since August 2020, Statistics Canada has sought out other countries for textile materials to manufacture all personal protective equipment. Canada's textile imports from the United States dropped from 53% in 2019 to 3.3% in 2020, with 90.7% of textiles coming from China in 2020. Canada's exports of face and eye protection has decreased between 3%-5% in order to secure medical supplies from their own citizens (Boushey, 2020). While countries are focused on their own vaccine progress and resources, we can still see instances of international cooperation during the COVID-19 pandemic. On March 13th, 2020, a team of scientists and medical experts were sent from China to Italy in order to help combat rising COVID-19 cases. The two countries teamed experts to implement stricter systems in Italy for social distancing and isolation. China also sent masks and medical supplies to Italy. Russia also assisted Italy in May 2020 by sending in virologists, medical equipment and pharmaceuticals. Additionally, Cuba sent Ebola virus experts to Italy for COVID-19 expertise, and the United States supplied the country with medical supplies (Poggioli, 2020). Overall, international relationships are on a delicate balance during the pandemic. Countries must make sure that they have enough vaccine shares for themselves, while contributing to the funding and negotiations of non-profit organizations that continue to carry out centuries of humanitarian efforts for all countries.

Chapter 16 - How Does It End?

By: Ivy Quan

Since the first case of the SARS-CoV-2 outbreak in Wuhan, China in November of 2019, countries, researchers, and pharmaceutical manufacturers have hastened to respond. World leaders have scrambled to enforce extensive public health measures in a desperate attempt to slow the pandemic until a vaccine is developed. Researchers have raced to develop and test their vaccine candidates, while media sites have broadcasted continual updates on promising vaccines, giving hope that a working vaccine will be available within 12-18 months. The entire world is relying on a safe and effective vaccine as a means to resume normal life, and this mounting pressure to develop a working vaccine has yielded remarkable vaccine development efforts. Due to the time pressure, most vaccine candidates are being developed with accelerated timelines and have started manufacturing prior to licensure. With immense private and public funding, there are hundreds of vaccine candidates being developed with many novel technologies such as nucleic acid and adenovirus vector vaccines. The unprecedented speed, volume, and innovation of COVID-19 vaccine development has been a source of hope that the end of the pandemic is near. To understand why mass immunization is our best strategy against COVID-19, we must first discuss several potential methods that can be used to combat disease outbreaks.

Let it Burn

There are three main strategies used to fight against pandemics, the first of which is waiting for natural herd immunity to develop. Since this method is similar to letting a fire burn itself out, we will refer to this strategy as "letting it burn". Herd immunity, while usually being associated with mass vaccination, can also occur when a majority of people develop immunity from the actual virus. The idea is, if most people in a certain population get infected, they will become immune to the pathogen and prevent transmission of the virus to those who have yet to be infected. During the early phases of the COVID-19 pandemic, the United Kingdom seemed to plan on taking this approach. By early March, when the outbreak was beginning to tear through parts of Europe, the inaction by the U.K. government contrasted the stringent restrictions being enforced by surrounding European countries. In many interviews, Sir Patrick Vallance, the U.K.'s Chief Scientific Advisor, stated that approximately 60% of their population would need to be infected in order to achieve herd immunity, in which the recovered patients can protect others by decreasing risk of transmission (Hunter, 2020). Their plan was to gradually suppress the outbreak to allow for 60% of their population to develop immunity, with the reason being that herd immunity would protect the U.K. population against the resurgence of a COVID-19 outbreak, which was expected in the winter of 2020. While it is possible that a population could be quickly protected against a pathogen if many people acquire immunity through infection, it will also inevitably result in a high death toll. Theoretically, if 60% of the U.K. gets infected, as per the government's former plans, out of a population of approximately 66.80 million people, around 40 million people would be infected ("United Kingdom population," 2020). If we factor in the case fatality rate for COVID-19, which is estimated to be around 14% for the U.K. as of August 2020, around 5.6 million people would die (Oke & Heneghan, 2020). To give context for these numbers, as of August 7, 2020, there have been approximately 718,000 deaths world-wide (Elfein, 2020). The estimated number of deaths in the U.K does not even account for the inescapable health care system collapse as the influx of COVID-19 cases overwhelm hospitals. If countries "let the fire burn itself out", the fire will burn quickly and mercilessly, and will leave a path of destruction behind it. Fortunately, the U.K. government quickly began enforcing stricter public health measures a couple weeks into March, including ordering the closure of non-essential businesses. However, their delayed response was largely criticized as being too little too late as COVID-19 ravaged through the U.K. just a week after they began enforcing stricter lockdowns. By the time the U.K. decided they wanted to put out the fire, it had already grown too large.

<u>Stamp Out the Fire</u>

The public lockdowns and social distancing eventually encouraged by the U.K. government are a couple of techniques comprising the second main strategy that we will refer to as "stamping out the fire". This strategy involves relying solely on social measures, such as placing restrictions on gatherings, enforcing isolation, closing non-essential services, and implementing aggressive testing and contact tracing. These techniques are analogous to stamping out a fire because the rigorous social measures deprive the fire of the fuel it needs to burn. If everyone in a population engaged in social distancing and those who test positive are quickly isolated until they recover, transmissibility rates would be low since the virus would not be able to effectively travel from host to host. While this sounds much less risky than "letting it burn", it also comes with some caveats. To work effectively, public health leaders must enforce restrictions early-on, before the fire grows too large to stamp out. This also requires the coordination of all people in areas of risk. In a pandemic, this means the entire globe. Let's take a look at how this strategy played during the 2003 SARS epidemic to judge the feasibility of stamping out COVID-19.

Overcoming the SARS epidemic of 2003 is widely lauded as a great public health victory because of the swift precautions taken by affected countries. Outside of East Asia, there were large outbreaks in Canada and the United States, each country having confirmed 250 and 75 cases respectively (World Health Organization, 2003). The WHO quickly advised all countries to avoid non-essential travel to high-risk locations, with the CDC and Health Canada also issuing their own travel alerts for countries with SARS outbreaks. Quarantine staff met planes and boats coming into the U.S. from China, Singapore, or Vietnam to contain any incoming infection risk. In Vietnam and Singapore, health officials used rigorous contact tracing to enforce quarantine upon suspected cases of SARS and all their contacts (Knobler et al., 2004). By acting quickly, both Vietnam and Singapore were successful in disrupting contact chains and containing a majority of the outbreak. Approximately eight months after the appearance of the first SARS cases, the WHO announced that the SARS Outbreak was contained globally (Centers for Disease Control and Prevention, 2013). These public health measures were originally adopted during the SARS outbreak to reduce transmission and buy time for the development of a vaccine. However, with a rapid, well-coordinated response and some luck, the virus was eliminated before a vaccine could be developed.

Similarly, in response to COVID-19, world leaders enforced social and travel restrictions with the intention to slow down transmission until a viable vaccine could be developed. However, if we exercised similar precautions during the COVID-19 pandemic as we did during the SARS epidemic, why haven't we been able to contain COVID-19 as quickly? There are several characteristic differences between SARS-CoV and SARS-CoV-2 that suggest why containing the 2019 SARS-CoV-2 pandemic may be more challenging. Although both viruses are transmitted through droplets, SARS-CoV-2 is a more transmissible virus and can therefore spread more easily and rapidly. Additionally, the incubation period–the amount of time between exposure and onset of symptoms–was estimated to be 2-7 days for SARS-CoV in contrast to the 14 day incubation period of SARS-CoV-2 (Centers for Disease Control and Prevention, 2005). Contact tracing is easier for viruses with shorter incubation periods because the risk of asymptomatic carriers is lower. The transmissibility and incubation period of SARS-CoV-2 makes COVID-19 more difficult to stamp out than SARS.

Despite these challenges, New Zealand and South Korea were able to contain most of the COVID-19 outbreak by acting quickly and decisively. On February 2, 2020, a mere 3 days after the WHO declared the coronavirus outbreak an international concern, New Zealand announced their first travel bans on incoming travellers from mainland China (World Health Organization, 2020a). They increased their restrictions on travel and social gatherings in the following weeks. South Korea also responded with haste; one week after their first COVID-19 case, companies were developing test kits and preparing for mass production (Thompson, 2020). Both New Zealand and South Korea implemented mass testing, stringent physical distancing, and contact tracing early into the outbreak. In particular, South Korea enforced meticulous contact tracing. After being ravaged by MERS in 2015, the country rewrote part of their legislation to allow health authorities free access to CCTV surveillance footage and cellular geolocation data during a health crisis (Thompson, 2020).

As a result, health officials were quickly able to identify who had potentially been exposed to COVID-19, and could instruct those contacts to self-isolate. While some may see this as a privacy violation, the tradeoff between privacy and public health could be justified by their enhanced ability to contact trace during a global health crisis. With their quick and decisive actions, New Zealand and South Korea were mostly able to contain their outbreaks. New Zealand was considered COVID-19 free on June 8, 2020 after a lack of reported new cases for 17 days, but unfortunately received new cases on June 14, 2020 when two travellers returned from the U.K. ("New Zealand lifts," 2020; Reuters, 2020). In August 2020, South Korea averaged approximately 40 new cases per day, a large portion of which are imported cases (Ministry of Health and Welfare of South Korea, 2020).

This demonstrates that while COVID-19 outbreaks can be contained in select countries that acted quickly, the global pandemic cannot be stamped out by implementing strict public health measures unless all countries collectively contain their outbreaks simultaneously.

Developing Fire Resistance

Mass immunization, the third strategy, involves developing and distributing a safe and effective vaccine. Using this method, enough of a population will gain immunity from the vaccine to achieve herd immunity. This will protect those in the immunized community who cannot receive the vaccine. If a disease outbreak is analogous to a wildfire, vaccination would be analogous to developing fire resistance. If all the trees in a forest were to become fire resistant, the wildfire cannot run rampant. With COVID-19, immunization is our most promising solution, as the other two strategies are either too risky or too challenging. While "letting it burn" theoretically works and would be a quick way to end an outbreak, the consequent death toll is alarming and the sudden influx of infection cases would overwhelm health care systems. On the other hand, "stamping it out" has potential to eliminate an outbreak while minimizing casualties. However, if we rely solely on this strategy, it must be adopted early in the outbreak by all affected countries. Its implementation during the COVID-19 pandemic would require effective, global collaboration to smother all the patches of fire at once, which is challenging. Vaccination also has its own caveats; the development of a viable vaccine can take a long time, and equitable distribution of a vaccine is difficult. Therefore, although "stamping it out" is ineffective on its own, implementing social restrictions is integral in minimizing transmission while vaccines are being developed and tested.

Upon administration of vaccines, it may be tempting to lift restrictions quickly and return to normal life. However, vaccination is not the silver bullet many people expect it to be. As discussed previously, early vaccine shortages will result in challenges with vaccine distribution both nationally and internationally. Additionally, the U.S. Food and Drug Administration's guidelines state that they expect a viable vaccine to have at least 50% efficacy (U.S. Food & Drug Administration, 2020). This means that a vaccine will be considered efficacious enough if it protects at least half of those immunized. However, researchers predict that at least 60% of the population must be protected to achieve herd immunity for COVID-19, so even though a vaccine is an integral tool to protect many people, it may not be able to end the pandemic alone (Bartsch et al., 2020). Distribution challenges and the potential lack of herd immunity indicate the need to maintain social measures even after vaccines have been administered. With the development and equitable distribution of a vaccine in conjunction with vigilant social distancing measures, we can effectively end the pandemic whilst minimizing casualties.

Throughout this book we saw how creative solutions and innovation can emerge from crisis. Combined or staggered trials together with early vaccine manufacturing have accelerated vaccine development and production to an unprecedented rate. Additionally, new vaccine platforms such as nucleic acid and adenovirus vector vaccines are in clinical trials for the first time and are some of the front-running vaccine candidates. These creative and novel aspects of vaccine development have pushed the world closer to overcoming the pandemic, and will undoubtedly shape our perception of what is possible with vaccines. Above all, we have seen how collaboration and patience are indispensable during a global health crisis. Citizens, public health officials, researchers, world leaders, and vaccine manufacturers need to work collectively to develop, test, and distribute a vaccine while maintaining proper social measures. We need patience and partnership, from knowledge to needle, so we can guide the world out of the COVID-19 pandemic.

References

14 Diseases You Almost Forgot About (Thanks to Vaccines). Centerss for Disease Control and Prevention. https://www.cdc.gov/vaccines/parents/diseases/forgot-14-diseases.html

Alberts B, Johnson A, Lewis J, et al. Molecular Biology of the Cell. 4th edition. New York: Garland Science; 2002. Chapter 24, The Adaptive Immune System. Available from: https://www.ncbi.nlm.nih.gov/books/NBK21070/

Apheresis. (n.d.). Retrieved August 8, 2020, from http://www.bcchildrens.ca/health-info/coping-support/cancer/apheresis

AstraZeneca takes next steps towards broad and equitable access to Oxford University's COVID-19 vaccine. (2020, June 04). Astrazeneca. https://www.astrazeneca.com/media-centre/press-releases/2020/astrazeneca-takes-next-steps-towards-broad-and-equitable-access-to-oxford-universitys-covid-19-vaccine.html

AstraZeneca to supply Europe with up to 400 million doses of Oxford University's vaccine at no profit. (2020, June 13). AstraZeneca. https://www.astrazeneca.com/content/astraz/media-centre/press-releases/2020/astrazeneca-to-supply-europe-with-up-to-400-million-doses-of-oxford-universitys-vaccine-at-no-profit.html.

Ballard, E. (1868). *On Vaccination, Its Value and Alleged Dangers*. Longmans.

Bao, L., Deng, W., Gao, H., Xiao, C., Liu, J., Xue, J., Lv, Q., Liu, J., Yu, P., Xu, Y., Qi, F., Qu, Y., Li, F., Xiang, Z., Yu, H., Gong, S., Liu, M., Wang, G., Wang, S., … Qin, C. (2020). Lack of Reinfection in Rhesus Macaques Infected with SARS-CoV-2. https://doi.org/10.1101/2020.03.13.990226

Bartsch, S. M., O'shea, K. J., Ferguson, M. C., Bottazzi, M. E., Wedlock, P. T., Strych, U., McKinnell, J. A., Siegmund, S. S., Cox, S. N., Hotez, P. J., Lee, B. Y. (2020). Vaccine Efficacy Needed for a COVID-19 Coronavirus Vaccine to Prevent or Stop an Epidemic as the Sole Intervention. *American Journal of Preventive Medicine*. https://doi.org/10.1016/j.amepre.2020.06.011

Belongia, E. A., & Naleway, A. L. (2003). Smallpox Vaccine: The Good, the Bad, and the Ugly. *Clinical Medicine & Research*, *1*(2), 87–92. https://doi.org/10.3121/cmr.1.2.87

Berkley, S. (2020, June 26*). What is the COVAX pillar, why do we need it and how will it work?*. Gavi The Vaccine Alliance. https://www.gavi.org/vaccineswork/gavi-ceo-dr-seth-berkley-explains-covax-pillar

BioPharma. (2014, August 4). *Use of freeze-drying in the stabilization of vaccines – Biopharma R&D Consultancy & Analytical Lab Services*. Biopharma RD Consultancy Analytical Lab Services. https://biopharma.co.uk/intelligent-freeze-drying/use-of-freeze-drying-in-the-stabilisation-of-vaccines/.

Blakney, A. K., McKay, P. F., Yus, B. I., Aldon, Y., & Shattock, R. J. (2019, July 12). Inside out: optimization of lipid nanoparticle formulations for exterior complexation and in vivo delivery of saRNA. *Gene Therapy*, *26*, 363-372. http://doi.org/10.1038/s41434-019-0095-2

Bloch, E. M., Shoham, S., Casadevall, A., Sachais, B. S., Shaz, B., Winters, J. L., van Buskirk, C., Grossman, B. J., Joyner, M., Henderson, J. P., Pekosz, A., Lau, B., Wesolowski, A., Katz, L., Shan, H., Auwaerter, P. G., Thomas, D., Sullivan, D. J., Paneth, N., … Tobian, A. A. R. (2020). Deployment of convalescent plasma for the prevention and treatment of COVID-19. *Journal of Clinical Investigation*, *130*(6), 2757-. Gale Academic OneFile.

Boseley, S. (2020a, July 3). *'I'm cautiously optimistic': Imperial's Robin Shattock on his coronavirus vaccine*. The Guardian. https://www.theguardian.com/society/2020/jul/03/im-cautiously-optimistic-imperials-robin-shattock-on-his-coronavirus-vaccine?utm_source=dlvr.it&utm_medium=twitter

Boseley, S. (2020b, June 30). *US secures world stock of key Covid-19 drug remdesivir*. The Guardian. https://www.theguardian.com/us-news/2020/jun/30/us-buys-up-world-stock-of-key-covid-19-drug

Boushey, N. (2020, August 5). *Trade in medical and protective goods, June 2020*. Statistics Canada. https://www150.statcan.gc.ca/n1/pub/45-28-0001/2020001/article/00061-eng.htm.

Brown, B. L., & McCullough, J. (2020). Treatment for emerging viruses: Convalescent plasma and COVID-19. *Transfusion and Apheresis Science*, *59*(3), 102790. https://doi.org/10.1016/j.transci.2020.102790

Callaway, E. (2020). Hundreds of people volunteer to be infected with coronavirus. *Nature*. https://doi.org/10.1038/d41586-020-01179-x

Centers for Disease Control and Prevention. (2005, May 3). *Frequently asked questions about SARS*. Centers for Disease Control and Prevention. https://www.cdc.gov/sars/about/faq.html

Centers for Disease Control and Prevention. (2009, July 29). *CDC advisors make recommendations for use of vaccine against novel H1N1*. Centers for Disease Control and Prevention. https://www.cdc.gov/media/pressrel/2009/r090729b.htm

Centers for Disease Control and Prevention. (2011, April 22). *Rotavirus Vaccine (Rotashield) and Intussusception.* Centers for Disease Control and Prevention. https://www.cdc.gov/vaccines/vpd-vac/rotavirus/vac-rotashield-historical.htm

Centers for Disease Control and Prevention. (2013, April 26). *CDC SARS Response Timeline.* Centers for Disease Control and Prevention. Retrieved from https://www.cdc.gov/about/history/sars/timeline.htm

Centers for Disease Control and Prevention. (2017, July 12). *Vaccine Basics.* Centers for Disease Control and Prevention. https://www.cdc.gov/smallpox/vaccine-basics/index.html.

Centers for Disease Control and Prevention. (2018, October 24). *Adjuvants help vaccines work better.* Centers for Disease Control and Prevention. https://www.cdc.gov/vaccinesafety/concerns/adjuvants.html.

Centers for Disease Control and Prevention. (2019, September 18). *Influenza Vaccination: A Summary for Clinicians.* Centers for Disease Control and Prevention. https://www.cdc.gov/flu/professionals/vaccination/vax-summary.htm.

Centers for Disease Control and Prevention. (2020, January 22). *Diphtheria, Tetanus, and Whooping Cough Vaccination: What Everyone Should Know.* Centers for Disease Control and Prevention. https://www.cdc.gov/vaccines/vpd/dtap-tdap-td/public/index.htm.

Chase, A., (1982). *A Human and Scientific Account of the Long and Continuing Struggle to Eradicate Infectious Diseases by Vaccination.* William Morrow.

Chokshi, D. A., & Kesselheim, A. S. (2008). Rethinking global access to vaccines. *Bmj, 336*(7647), 750–753. https://doi.org/10.1136/bmj.39497.598044.be

Clem, A. S. (2011). Fundamentals of vaccine immunology. *Journal of Global Infectious Diseases, 3*(1), 73. https://doi.org/10.4103/0974-777X.77299

Cohen , J. (2020, April 23). *COVID-19 vaccine protects monkeys from new coronavirus, Chinese biotech reports.* Science. https://www.sciencemag.org/news/2020/04/covid-19-vaccine-protects-monkeys-new-coronavirus-chinese-biotech-reports.

Copeman, S.M. (1899). *Vaccination, Its Natural History and Pathology.* Macmillan. deBary, W.T. (Ed.). (1972). *The Buddhist Tradition in India. China and Japan.* Vintage Books.

DeStefano, F., & Shimabukuro, T. T. (2019). The MMR Vaccine and Autism. *Annual Review of Virology, 6*(1), 585–600. https://doi.org/10.1146/annurev-virology-092818-015515

Dong, E., Du, H., & Gardner, L. (2020). An interactive web-based dashboard to track COVID-19 in real time. *The Lancet Infectious Diseases, 20*(5), 533–534. https://doi.org/10.1016/s1473-3099(20)30120-1

Doremalen, N. V., Haddock, E., Feldmann, F., Meade-White, K., Bushmaker, T., Fischer, R. J., Okumura, A., Hanley, P. W., Saturday, G., Edwards, N. J., Clark, M. H. A., Lambe, T., Gilbert, S. C., Munster, V. J. (2020a, June 10). A single dose of ChAdOx1 MERS provides protective immunity in rhesus macaques. *Science Advances, 6*(24). http://doi.org/10.1126/sciadv.aba8399

Doremalen, N. V., Lambe, T., Spencer, A., Belij-Rammerstorfer, S., Purushotham, J. N., Port, J. R., … Munster, V. J. (2020b). ChAdOx1 nCoV-19 vaccination prevents SARS-CoV-2 pneumonia in rhesus macaques. https://doi.org/10.1101/2020.05.13.093195

Edwards, K. M. (2005). Overview of Pertussis. *The Pediatric*

Infectious Disease Journal, 24(Supplement). https://doi. org/10.1097/01.inf.0000166154.47013.47

Elfein, J. (2020, August 7). *Number of novel coronavirus (COVID-19) deaths worldwide as of August 7, 2020, by country.* Statista. https://www.statista.com/statistics/1093256/novel-coronavirus-2019ncov-deaths-worldwide-by-country/

Enders, J.F., Weller, T.H., Robbins, F.C. (1949). *Cultivation of the Lansing strain of poliomyelitis virus in culture of various human embryonic tissues.* Science.

Erman, M., & Banerjee, A. (2020, July 22). *Pfizer signs deal with U.S. for 100 million coronavirus vaccine doses.* The Globe and Mail. https://www.theglobeandmail.com/business/international-business/us-business/article-pfizer-has-signed-deal-with-us-for-100-million-coronavirus-vaccine/

Estimated Incubation Period of COVID-19. (n.d.). American College of Cardiology. Retrieved August 8, 2020, from http%3a%2f%2fwww.acc.org%2flatest-in-cardiology%2fjournal-scans%2f2020%2f05%2f11%2f15%2f18%2fthe-incubation-period-of-coronavirus-disease

Felter, C. (2020, July 23). *What Is the World Doing to Create a COVID-19 Vaccine?.* Council on Foreign Relations. https://www.cfr.org/backgrounder/what-world-doing-create-covid-19-vaccine.

Folegatti, P. M., Bittaye, M., Flaxman, M., Lopez, F. R., Bellamy, D., Kupke, A., Mair, C., Makinson, R., Sheridan, J., Rohde, C., Halwe, S., Jeong, Y., Park, Y., Kim, J., Song, M., Boyd, A., Tran, N., Silman, D., Poulton, I., … Gilbert, S. (2020a, July 1). Safety and immunogenicity of a candidate Middle East respiratory syndrome coronavirus viral-vectored vaccine: a dose-escalation, open-label, non-randomised, uncontrolled, phase 1 trial. *The Lancet Infectious Diseases, 20*(7), 816-826. http://doi.org/10.1016/S1473-3099(20)30160-2

Folegatti, P. M., Ewer, K. J., Aley, P. K., Angus, B., Becker, S., Belij-Rammerstorfer, S., Bellamy, D., Bibi, S., Bittaye,

M., Clutterbuck, E. A., Dold, C., Faust, S. N., Finn, A., Flaxman, A. L., Hallis, B., Heath, P., Jenkin, D., Lazarus, R., Makinson, R., … Pollard, A. J. (2020b). Safety and immunogenicity of the ChAdOx1 nCoV-19 vaccine against SARS-CoV-2: a preliminary report of a phase 1/2, single-blind, randomised controlled trial. *The Lancet*. https://doi.org/10.1016/s0140-6736(20)31604-4

Gao, Q., Bao, L., Mao, H., Wang, L., Xu, K., Yang, M., Li, Y., Zhu, L., Wang, N., Lv, Z., Gao, H., Ge, X., Kan, B., Hu, Y., Liu, J., Cai, F., Jiang, D., Yin, Y., Qin, C., … Qin, C. (2020). Development of an inactivated vaccine candidate for SARS-CoV-2. *Science*, *369*(6499), 77–81. https://doi.org/10.1126/science.abc1932

Garner-Spitzer, E., Wagner, A., Paulke-Korinek, M., Kollaritsch, H., Heinz, F. X., Redlberger-Fritz, M., Stiasny, K., Fischer, G. F., Kundi, M., Wiedermann, U. (2013). Tick-Borne Encephalitis (TBE) and Hepatitis B Nonresponders Feature Different Immunologic Mechanisms in Response to TBE and Influenza Vaccination with Involvement of Regulatory T and B Cells and IL-10. *The Journal of Immunology*, *191*(5), 2426–2436. https://doi.org/10.4049/jimmunol.1300293

Gavi announces 75 countries intend to join COVAX access facility. (2020, July 16). Pharmaceutical Technology. https://www.pharmaceutical-technology.com/news/covax-facility-covid-vaccines-access/

Gavi launches innovative financing mechanism for access to COVID-19 vaccines. (2020, June 4). Gavi The Vaccine Alliance. https://www.gavi.org/news/media-room/gavi-launches-innovative-financing-mechanism-access-covid-19-vaccines

Gavi. *More than 150 countries engaged in COVID-19 vaccine global access facility.* (2020, July 15). Gavi, the Vaccine Alliance. https://www.gavi.org/news/media-room/more-150-countries-engaged-covid-19-vaccine-global-access-facility.

Gellin, B. (2020). Why vaccine rumours stick—and getting them unstuck. *The Lancet, 396*(10247), 303–304. https://doi.org/10.1016/s0140-6736(20)31640-8

Government of Canada. (2019, December 11*). Canadian adverse events following immunization surveillance system (CAEFISS).* Government of Canada. https://www.canada.ca/en/public-health/services/immunization/canadian-adverse-events-following-immunization-surveillance-system-caefiss.html

Gowrisankar, A., Rondoni, L., & Banerjee, S. (2020). Can India develop herd immunity against COVID-19? *The European Physical Journal Plus, 135*(6). https://doi.org/10.1140/epjp/s13360-020-00531-4

Gursel, M., & Gursel, I. (2020). Is global BCG vaccination-induced trained immunity relevant to the progression of SARS-CoV-2 pandemic? *Allergy, 75*(7), 1815–1819. https://doi.org/10.1111/all.14345

Halstead, S. B., Mahalingam, S., Marovich, M. A., Ubol, S., & Mosser, D. M. (2010). Intrinsic antibody-dependent enhancement of microbial infection in macrophages: disease regulation by immune complexes. *The Lancet Infectious Diseases, 10*(10), 712–722. https://doi.org/10.1016/s1473-3099(10)70166-3

Hamilton, I. A. (2020, April 6). *Bill Gates is funding 7 new factories for potential coronavirus vaccines.* World Economic Forum. https://www.weforum.org/agenda/2020/04/bill-gates-7-potential-coronavirus-vaccines.

Herd immunity and COVID-19 (coronavirus): What you need to know. (n.d.). Mayo Clinic. Retrieved August 9, 2020, from https://www.mayoclinic.org/diseases-conditions/coronavirus/in-depth/herd-immunity-and-coronavirus/art-20486808

Hinman, A. R., Orenstein, W. A., & Mortimer, E. A. (1992). When, where, and how do immunizations fail? *Annals of Epidemiology*, *2*(6), 805–812. https://doi.org/10.1016/1047-2797(92)90074-z

Hopkins, J. (2020). *The Immune System*. https://www.hopkinsmedicine.org/health/conditions-and-diseases/the-immune-system.

Hotez, P. J. (2014). *"Vaccine Diplomacy": Historical Perspectives and Future Directions*, *8*(6). https://doi.org/10.1371/journal.pntd.0002808

How Vaccines Work. (2019, November 22). PublicHealth. org. https://www.publichealth.org/public-awareness/understanding-vaccines/vaccines-work/.

Hudgens, M. G., Gilbert, P. B., & Self, S. G. (2004, April 13). Endpoints in vaccine trials. *Statistical Methods in Medical Research*, *13*(2), 89-114. http://doi.org/10.1191/0962280204sm356ra

Huneycutt, B., Lurie, N., Rotenburg, S., Wilder, R., & Hatchett, R. (2020, February 24). Finding equipoise: CEPI revises its equitable access policy. *Elsevier*, 38(9), 2144-2148. http://doi.org/10.1016/j.vaccine.2019.12.055

Hunter, D. J. (2020, April 16). Covid-19 and the stiff upper lip - the pandemic response in the United Kingdom. *The New England Journal of Medicine*, 382(e31). http://doi.org/10.1056/NEJMp2005755

INOVIO announces positive interim phase 1 data for INO-4800 vaccine for COVID-19. (2020, June 30). Cision PR Newswire. https://www.prnewswire.com/news-releases/inovio-announces-positive-interim-phase-1-data-for-ino-4800-vaccine-for-covid-19-301085537.html

Institute of Medicine (US) Committee on the Evaluation of
Vaccine Purchase Financing in the United States. Financing
Vaccines in the 21st Century: Assuring Access and Availability.
Washington (DC): National Academies Press (US); 2003. 4,
Delivery Systems. Available from: https://www.ncbi.nlm.nih.gov/
books/NBK221821/

International Labour Organization. (2020, June 30). *ILO Monitor:
COVID-19 and the world of work. 5th edition.* World
Health Organization. https://www.ilo.org/global/topics/
coronavirus/impacts-and-responses/WCMS_749399/lang--
en/index.htm

Iwasaki, A., & Yang, Y. (2020). The potential danger of
suboptimal antibody responses in COVID-19. *Nature
Reviews Immunology, 20*(6), 339–341. https://doi.
org/10.1038/s41577-020-0321-6

Jackson, L. A., Anderson, E. J., Rouphael, N. G., Roberts, P. C.,
Makhene, M., Coler, R. N., McCullough, M. P., Chappell,
J. .D., Denison, M. R., Stevens, L. J., Pruijssers, A. J.,
McDermott, A., Flach, B., Doria-Rose, N. A., Corbett, K.
S., Morabito, K. M., O'Dell, S., Schmidt, S. D., Swanson,
P. A., … Beigel, J. H. (2020). An mRNA Vaccine against
SARS-CoV-2 - Preliminary Report. *New England Journal
of Medicine.* https://doi.org/10.1056/nejmoa2022483

Jamrozik, E., & Selgelid, M. J. (2020). COVID-19 human
challenge studies: ethical issues. *The Lancet Infectious
Diseases, 20*(8). https://doi.org/10.1016/s1473-
3099(20)30438-2

Khamsi, R. (2020, April 9). *If a coronavirus vaccine arrives,
can the world make enough?* Nature News. https://www.

nature.com/articles/d41586-020-01063-8.

Khan, K. H. (2013, March 1). DNA vaccines: roles against
diseases. *Germs*, *3*(1), 26-35. http://doi.org/10.11599/
germs.2013.1034

Khanal, S., Ghimire, P., & Dhamoon, A. (2018). The
Repertoire of Adenovirus in Human Disease: The Innocuous
to the Deadly. *Biomedicines*, *6*(1), 30. https://doi.org/10.3390/
biomedicines6010030

Knobler, S., Mahmoud, A., Lemon, S., Mack, A., Sivitz, L., &
Oberholtzer, K. (2004). *Learning from SARS: Preparing for the
next disease outbreak: Workshop summary*. Washington, DC:
National Academies Press. http://doi.org/10.17226/10915

Knudson, C. M., & Jackson, J. B. (2020). COVID-19 convalescent
plasma: Phase 2. *Transfusion*, *60*(6), 1332–1333. https://doi.
org/10.1111/trf.15842

Krishnakumar, R., & Blelloch, R. H. (2013). Epigenetics
of cellular reprogramming. *Current Opinion in Genetics
& Development*, *23*(5), 548–555. https://doi.org/10.1016/j.
gde.2013.06.005

Krugman, S. (1983). Further-Attenuated Measles Vaccine:
Characteristics and Use. *Clinical Infectious Diseases*, *5*(3), 477–
481. https://doi.org/10.1093/clinids/5.3.477

Kupferschmidt, K. (2020, July 29). *'Vaccine nationalism'
threatens global plan to distribute COVID-19 shots fairly*.
Science. https://www.sciencemag.org/news/2020/07/vaccine-
nationalism-threatens-global-plan-distribute-covid-19-shots-fairly.

La Vignera, S., Cannarella, R., Condorelli, R. A., Torre, F.,
Aversa, A., & Calogero, A. E. (2020). Sex-Specific SARS-CoV-2
Mortality: Among Hormone-Modulated ACE2 Expression,
Risk of Venous Thromboembolism and Hypovitaminosis D.
International Journal of Molecular Sciences, *21*(8). https://doi.
org/10.3390/ijms21082948

Lai, J., Ma, S., Wang, Y., Cai, Z., Hu, J., Wei, N., Wu, J., Du, H.,
Chen, T., Li, R., Tan, H., Kang, L., Yao, L., Huang, M., Wang,
H., Wang, G., Liu, Z., Hu, S. (2020). Factors Associated With
Mental Health Outcomes Among Health Care Workers Exposed to
Coronavirus Disease 2019. *JAMA Network Open*, *3*(3). https://doi.

org/10.1001/jamanetworkopen.2020.3976

Le, T. T., Andreadakis, Z., Kumar, A., Román, R. G., Tollefsen, S., Saville, M., & Mayhew, S. (2020). The COVID-19 vaccine development landscape. *Nature Reviews Drug Discovery, 19*(5), 305–306. https://doi.org/10.1038/d41573-020-00073-5

Lechardeur, D., Sohn, K., Haardt, M., Joshi, P. B., Monck, M., Graham, R. W., Beatty, B., Squire, J., O'Brodovich, H., Lukacs, G. L. (1999, April 17). Metabolic instability of plasmid DNA in the cytosol: a potential barrier to gene transfer. *Gene Therapy, 6*, 482-497. http://doi.org/10.1038/sj.gt.3300867

Letter from James E. Clyburn, Chairman, Select Subcommittee on the Coronavirus Crisis, and Carolyn B. Maloney, Chairwoman, Committee on Oversight and Reform, to Alex M. Azar II, Secretary, Department of Health and Human Services (June 2, 2020). https://oversight.house.gov/sites/democrats.oversight. house.gov/files/2020-06-02.Clyburn%20CBM%20to%20 HHS%20re%20Vaccine%20and%20Treatment%20Contracts.pdf

Leung, A.K. (1996). *Variolation and vaccination in late imperial China, ca 1570-1911*. Elsevier.

Li, F. (2014). Receptor Recognition Mechanisms of Coronaviruses: A Decade of Structural Studies. *Journal of Virology, 89*(4), 1954–1964. https://doi.org/10.1128/JVI.02615-14

Li, G., Fan, Y., Lai, Y., Han, T., Li, Z., Zhou, P., Pan, P., Wang, W., Hu, D., Liu, X., Zhang, Q., & Wu, J. (2020). Coronavirus infections and immune responses. *Journal of Medical Virology, 92*(4), 424–432. https://doi.org/10.1002/jmv.25685

Liang, Y., Wang, M.-L., Chien, C.-S., Yarmishyn, A. A., Yang, Y.-P., Lai, W.-Y., Luo, Y. H., Lin, Y.-T., Chen, Y.-J., Chang, P.-C., Chiou, S.-H. (2020). Highlight of Immune Pathogenic Response and Hematopathologic Effect in SARS-CoV, MERS-CoV, and SARS-Cov-2 Infection. *Frontiers in Immunology, 11*. https://doi.org/10.3389/fimmu.2020.01022

Liu, M. A. (2019, April 24). A comparison of plasmid DNA and mRNA as vaccine technologies. *Vaccines, 7*(2), 37. http://

doi.org/10.3390/vaccines7020037

Lloyd-Smith, J. O., George, D., Pepin, K. M., Pitzer, V. E., Pulliam, J. R. C., Dobson, A. P., Hudson, P. J., Grenfell, B. T. (2009). Epidemic Dynamics at the Human-Animal Interface. *Science*, *326*(5958), 1362–1367. https://doi.org/10.1126/science.1177345

Loveface, B. (2020, August 07). *Pfizer agrees to manufacture Gilead's coronavirus drug remdesivir*. CNBC. https://www.cnbc.com/2020/08/07/pfizer-agrees-to-manufacture-gileads-coronavirus-drug-remdesivir.html

Magnusson, S. E., Altenburg, A. F., Bengtsson, K. L., Bosman, F., Vries, R. D. D., Rimmelzwaan, G. F., & Stertman, L. (2018). Matrix-M™ adjuvant enhances immunogenicity of both protein- and modified vaccinia virus Ankara-based influenza vaccines in mice. *Immunologic Research*, *66*(2), 224–233. https://doi.org/10.1007/s12026-018-8991-x

Magritte, R. (1905). *«Those who cannot remember the past are condemned to repeat it.»--George Santayana, The Life of Reason, 1905. From the series Great Ideas of Western Man.* Smithsonian American Art Museum. https://americanart.si.edu/artwork/those-who-cannot-remember-past-are-condemned-repeat-it-george-santayana-life-reason-1905.

Mancini, D. P., Cookson, C., & Kuchler, H. (2020, July 28). *Moderna pitches virus vaccine at about $50-$60 per course.* Financial Times. https://www.ft.com/content/405c0d07-d15a-4f5b-8a77-3c2fbd5d4c1c

Marano, G., Vaglio, S., Pupella, S., Facco, G., Catalano, L., Liumbruno, G. M., & Grazzini, G. (2016). Convalescent plasma: New evidence for an old therapeutic tool? *Blood Transfusion*, *14*(2), 152–157. https://doi.org/10.2450/2015.0131-15

Mccarthy, K. A., Chabot-Couture, G., Famulare, M., Lyons, H. M., & Mercer, L. D. (2017). The risk of type 2 oral polio vaccine use in post-cessation outbreak response. *BMC Medicine*, *15*(1). https://doi.org/10.1186/s12916-017-0937-y

Mcgonagle, D., Sharif, K., O'regan, A., & Bridgewood, C. (2020). The Role of Cytokines including Interleukin-6 in COVID-19 induced Pneumonia and Macrophage Activation Syndrome-Like Disease. *Autoimmunity Reviews*, *19*(6), 102537. https://doi.org/10.1016/j.autrev.2020.102537

McKay, P. F., Hu, K., Blakney, A. K., Samnuan, K., Brown, J. C., Penn, R., ... Shattock, R. J. (2020, July 9). Self-amplifying RNA SARS-CoV-2 lipid nanoparticle vaccine candidate induces high neutralizing antibody titers in mice. *Nature Communications, 11.* http://doi.org/10.1038/s41467-020-17409-9

McKee, C., & Bohannon, K. (2016). Exploring the Reasons Behind Parental Refusal of Vaccines. *The Journal of Pediatric Pharmacology and Therapeutics : JPPT, 21*(2), 104–109. https://doi.org/10.5863/1551-6776-21.2.104

McKenna , M. (2010, April 26). *H1N1 LESSONS LEARNED Vaccine production foiled, confirmed experts' predictions.* CIDRAP. https://www.cidrap.umn.edu/news-perspective/2010/04/h1n1-lessons-learned-vaccine-production-foiled-confirmed -experts.

Miller, D., Martin, M. A., Harel, N., Kustin, T., Tirosh, O., Meir, M., Sorek, N., Gefen-Halvei, S., Amit, S., Vorontsov, O., Wolf, D., Peretz, A., Shemer-Avni, S., Roif-Kaminsky, D., Kopelman, N., Huppert, A., Koelle, K., Stern, A. (2020). Full genome viral sequences inform patterns of SARS-CoV-2 spread into and within Israel. https://doi.org/10.1101/2020.05.21.20104521

Ministry of Health and Welfare of South Korea. (2020). *Cases in Korea.* Coronavirus Disease, Republic of Korea. http://ncov.mohw.go.kr/en/bdBoardList.do?brdId=16&brdGubun=161&dataGubun=&ncvContSeq=&contSeq=&board_id=

Moderna's Work on a COVID-19 Vaccine Candidate | Moderna, Inc. (n.d.). Retrieved August 8, 2020, from https://www.modernatx.com/modernas-work-potential-vaccine-against-covid-19?utm_source=homepage&utm_medium=slider&utm_campaign=covid

Modjarrad, K., Lin, L., George, S. L., Stephenson, K. E., Eckels, K. H., Barrera, R. A. D. L., Jarman, R. G., Sondergaard, E., Tennant, J., Ansel, J. L., Mills, K., Koren, M., Robb, M. L., Barrett, J., Thompson, J., Kosel, A. E., Dawson, P., Hale, A., Tan, C. S., Michael, N. L. (2018). Preliminary aggregate safety and immunogenicity results from three trials of a purified inactivated Zika virus vaccine candidate: phase 1, randomised, double-blind, placebo-controlled clinical trials. *The Lancet, 391*(10120), 563–571. https://doi.org/10.1016/s0140-6736(17)33106-9

Montecino-Rodriguez, E., Berent-Maoz, B., & Dorshkind, K. (2013). Causes, consequences, and reversal of immune system aging. *Journal of Clinical Investigation, 123*(3), 958–965. https://doi.org/10.1172/jci64096

Moore, Z. S., Seward, J. F., & Lane, J. M. (2006). Smallpox. *The Lancet, 367*(9508), 425–435. https://doi.org/10.1016/s0140-6736(06)68143-9

National Institutes of Health. (2020a, July 14). *Potent antibodies found in people recovered from COVID-19.* National Institutes of Health. https://www.nih.gov/news-events/nih-research-matters/potent-antibodies-found-people-recovered-covid-19.

National Institutes of Health. (2020b, July 2). *Immune response: MedlinePlus Medical Encyclopedia.* MedlinePlus. https://medlineplus.gov/ency/article/000821.htm.

National Institutes of Health. (2020c, July 27). *Phase 3 clinical trial of investigational vaccine for COVID-19 begins.* National Institutes of Health. https://www.nih.gov/news-events/news-releases/phase-3-clinical-trial-investigational-vaccine-covid-19-begins.

Nature, E. (2020). Getting out of the World Health Organization Might Not Be as Easy as Trump Thinks. *Nature, 582*(7813), 459–459. https://doi.org/10.1038/d41586-020-01847-y

New Zealand lifts all Covid restrictions, declaring the nation virus-free. (2020, June 8). BBC News. https://www.bbc.com/news/world-asia-52961539

O'Neill, L. A. J., & Netea, M. G. (2020). BCG-induced trained immunity: can it offer protection against COVID-19? Nature Reviews Immunology, 20(6), 335–337. https://doi.org/10.1038/s41577-020-0337-y

Offit, P.A. (2005). *The Cutter Incident: How America's First Polio Vaccine Led to the Growing Vaccine Crisis.* Yale University Press.

O'Hare, R., & Wighton, K. (2020, June 15). *Imperial to begin first human trials of new COVID-19 vaccine.* Imperial College London. https://www.imperial.ac.uk/news/198314/imperial-begin-first-human-trials-covid-19/

Oke, J., & Heneghan, C. (2020, March 17). *Global Covid-19 case fatality rates.* CEBM. https://www.cebm.net/covid-19/global-covid-19-case-fatality-rates/

Omer, S. B., Malani, P., & Rio, C. D. (2020). The COVID-19 Pandemic in the US. *Jama.* https://doi.org/10.1001/jama.2020.5788

Padron-Regalado, E. (2020). Vaccines for SARS-CoV-2: Lessons from Other Coronavirus Strains. *Infectious Diseases and Therapy, 9*(2), 255–274. https://doi.org/10.1007/s40121-020-00300-x

Pagliusi, S., Jarrett, S., Hayman, B., Kreysa, U., Prasad, S. D., Reers, M., Thai, P. H., Wu, K., Zhang, Y. T., Baek, Y. O., Kumar, A., Evtushenko, A., Jadhav, S., Meng, W., Dat, D. T., Huang, W., Desai, S. (2020). Emerging manufacturers engagements in the COVID −19 vaccine research, development and supply. *Vaccine, 38*(34), 5418–5423. https://doi.org/10.1016/j.vaccine.2020.06.022

Parish, H.J. (1965). *A History of Immunization.* E & S Livingstone.

Pasteur, L., Chamberland, C-E., Roux, E. (1881). *Sur la vaccination charbonneuse.* C R Acad Sci Paris.

Pead, P.J. (2006) *Vaccination Rediscovered: New Light in the Dawn of Man's Quest for Immunity.* Timefile Books.

Pelčić, G., Karačić, S., Mikirtichan, G. L., Kubar, O. I., Leavitt, F. J., Cheng-tek Tai, M., Morishita, N., Vuletić, S., & Tomašević, L. (2016). Religious exception for vaccination or religious excuses for avoiding vaccination. *Croatian Medical Journal, 57*(5), 516–521. https://doi.org/10.3325/cmj.2016.57.516

People who are at high risk for severe illness from COVID-19. (2020, July 13). Government of Canada. https://www.canada.ca/en/public-health/services/publications/diseases-conditions/people-high-risk-for-severe-illness-covid-19.html

Petersen, E., Koopmans, M., Go, U., Hamer, D. H., Petrosillo, N., Castelli, F., Storgaard, M., Khalili, S. A., Simonsen, L. (2020). Comparing SARS-CoV-2 with SARS-CoV and influenza pandemics. *The Lancet Infectious Diseases.* https://doi.org/10.1016/s1473-3099(20)30484-9

Pfizer and BioNTech announce early positive update from German phase 1/2 COVID-19 vaccine study, including first T cell response data. (2020, July 20). Business Wire. https://www.businesswire.com/news/home/20200720005408/en/

Poggioli, S. (2020, March 25). *For Help On Coronavirus, Italy Turns To China, Russia And Cuba*. NPR. https://www.npr.org/sections/coronavirus-live-updates/2020/03/25/821345465/for-help-on-coronavirus-italy-turns-to-china-russia-and-cuba.

Pollack, A. (2015, September 20). *Drug Goes From $13.50 a Tablet to $750, Overnight*. The New York Times. https://www.nytimes.com/2015/09/21/business/a-huge-overnight-increase-in-a-drugs-price-raises-protests.html

Qin, E., Shi, H., Tang, L., Wang, C., Chang, G., Ding, Z., Zhoa, K., Wang, J., Chen, Z., Yu, M., Si, B., Liu, J., Wu, D., Cheng, X., Yang, B., Peng, W., Meng, Q., Liu, B., Han, W., … Zhu, Q. (2006). Immunogenicity and protective efficacy in monkeys of purified inactivated Vero-cell SARS vaccine. *Vaccine*, *24*(7), 1028–1034. https://doi.org/10.1016/j.vaccine.2005.06.038

Questions and Answers | Pandemic Influenza (Flu) | CDC. (2020, June 16). https://www.cdc.gov/flu/pandemic-resources/basics/faq.html

Rabaan, A. A., Al-Ahmed, S. H., Haque, S., Sah, R., Tiwari, R., Malik, Y. S., Dhama, K., Yatoo, M. I., Bonilla-Aldana, D. K., & Rodriguez-Morales, A. J. (n.d.). *SARS-CoV-2, SARS-CoV, and MERS-CoV: a comparative overview*. 11.

Rajendran, K., Krishnasamy, N., Rangarajan, J., Rathinam, J., Natarajan, M., & Ramachandran, A. (2020). Convalescent plasma transfusion for the treatment of COVID-19: Systematic review. *Journal of Medical Virology*, jmv.25961. https://doi.org/10.1002/jmv.25961

Redding, L., & Werner, D. B. (2009, September 8). DNA vaccines in veterinary use. *Expert Review of Vaccines*, *8*(9), 1251-1276. http://doi.org/10.1586/erv.09.77

Reuters, T. (2020, June 15). *New Zealand reports 2 news COVID-19 cases, days after declaring itself free of the coronavirus*. CBC . https://www.cbc.ca/news/world/new-zealand-covid-2-cases-1.5613516

Ricke, D., & Malone, R. W. (2020). Medical Countermeasures Analysis of 2019-nCoV and Vaccine Risks for Antibody-Dependent Enhancement (ADE). *SSRN Electronic Journal*. https://doi.org/10.2139/ssrn.3546070

Robbins, F.C., (2004). *The History of Polio Vaccine Development*. Saunders.

Rogers, J. (2020, July 23). *CEPI extends funding call to accelerate development and global manufacture of COVID-19 vaccines*. CEPI. https://cepi.net/news_cepi/cepi-extends-funding-call-to-accelerate-development-and-global-manufacture-of-covid-19-vaccines/.

Rogers, L. S., & Health, J. B. S. of P. (n.d.). *What is Herd Immunity and How Can We Achieve It With COVID-19?* Johns Hopkins Bloomberg School of Public Health. Retrieved August 9, 2020, from https://www.jhsph.edu/covid-19/articles/achieving-herd-immunity-with-covid19.html

Roser, M., Ritchie, H., Ortiz-Ospina, E., & Hasell, J. (2020, March 4). *Coronavirus Pandemic (COVID-19) - Statistics and Research*. Our World in Data. https://ourworldindata.org/coronavirus.

Rothan, H. A., & Byrareddy, S. N. (2020). The epidemiology and pathogenesis of coronavirus disease (COVID-19) outbreak. *Journal of Autoimmunity*, *109*, 102433. https://doi.org/10.1016/j.jaut.2020.102433

RTS,S Clinical Trials Partnership Members, . (2015, July 4). Efficacy and safety of RTS,S/AS01 malaria vaccine with or without a booster dose in infants and children in Africa: final results of a phase 3, individually randomized, controlled trial. *The Lancet*, *386*(9988), 31-45. http://doi.org/10.1016/S0140-6736(15)60721-8

Ruijs, W. L. M., Hautvast, J. L. A., van IJzendoorn, G., van Ansem, W. J. C., van der Velden, K., & Hulscher, M. E. (2012). How orthodox protestant parents decide on the vaccination of their children: A qualitative study. *BMC Public Health*, *12*(1), 408. https://doi.org/10.1186/1471-2458-12-408

Sanofi Statement on Zika Vaccine License. (2017, September 1). Sanofi. http://www.news.sanofi.us/press-statements?item=991.

Sardesai, N. Y., & Weiner, D. B. (2011, June). Electroporation delivery of DNA vaccines: prospects for success. *Current Opinion in Immunology*, *23*(3), 421-429. http://doi.org/10.1016/j.coi.2011.03.008

SARS | Frequently Asked Questions | CDC. (2019, February 8). Centers for Disease Control and Prevention. https://www.cdc.gov/sars/about/faq.html

Schaik, W. (2020). *Expert reaction to questions about COVID-19 and viral load*. Science Media Centre. https://www.sciencemediacentre.org/expert-reaction-to-questions-about-covid-19-and-viral-load/.

Schröder, I. (2020). COVID-19: A Risk Assessment Perspective. *ACS Chemical Health & Safety*, *27*(3), 160–169. https://doi.org/10.1021/acs.chas.0c00035

Seow, J., Graham, C., Merrick, B., Acors, S., Steel, K. J., Hemmings, O., O'Bryne, A., Kouphou, N., Pickering, S., Galao, R., Betancor, G., D'Wilson, H., Signell, A. W., Winstone, H., Kerridge, C., Temperton, N., Snell, L., Bisnauthsing, K,. Moore, A., … Doores, K. (2020). Longitudinal evaluation and decline of antibody responses in SARS-CoV-2 infection. https://doi.org/10.1101/2020.07.09.20148429

Sharp, P. M., & Hahn, B. H. (2011). Origins of HIV and the AIDS Pandemic. *Cold Spring Harbor Perspectives in Medicine*, *1*(1). https://doi.org/10.1101/cshperspect.a006841

Shereen, M. A., Khan, S., Kazmi, A., Bashir, N., & Siddique, R. (2020). COVID-19 infection: Origin, transmission, and characteristics of human coronaviruses. *Journal of*

Advanced Research, 24, 91–98. https://doi.org/10.1016/j.jare.2020.03.005

Sherman, I.W. (2006). *The Power of Plagues.* ASM Press.

Singh, K., & Mehta, S. (2016, January). The clinical development process for a novel preventive vaccine: An overview. *Journal of Postgraduate Medicine, 62*(1), 4-11. http://doi.org/10.4103/0022-3859.173187

Smith-Gill, S. J., Lavoie, T. B., & Mainhart, C. R. (1984). Antigenic regions defined by monoclonal antibodies correspond to structural domains of avian lysozyme. *Journal of immunology (Baltimore, Md. : 1950), 133*(1), 384–393.

Snyder, C. M., Begor, W., & Berndt, E. R. (2011). Economic Perspectives On The Advance Market Commitment For Pneumococcal Vaccines. *Health Affairs, 30*(8), 1508–1517. https://doi.org/10.1377/hlthaff.2011.0403

Spiro, T., & Emanuel, Z. (2020, July 28). *A Comprehensive COVID-19 Vaccine Plan.* Center for American Progress. https://www.americanprogress.org/issues/healthcare/reports/2020/07/28/488196/comprehensive-covid-19-vaccine-plan/.

Srinivasan, L., Harris, M. C., & Kilpatrick, L. E. (2017). Cytokines and Inflammatory Response in the Fetus and Neonate. *Fetal and Neonatal Physiology.* https://doi.org/10.1016/b978-0-323-35214-7.00128-1

Stanford Children's Health. (n.d.). Retrieved August 8, 2020, from https://www.stanfordchildrens.org/en/topic/default?id=what-is-plasma-160-37

Subbarao, K., & Mahanty, S. (2020). Respiratory Virus Infections: Understanding COVID-19. *Immunity, 52*(6), 905–909. https://doi.org/10.1016/j.immuni.2020.05.004

The Access to COVID-19 Tools (ACT) Accelerator. (n.d.). World Health Organization. https://www.who.int/initiatives/act-accelerator

The College of Physicians of Philadelphia. (2018, January 10). *The Future of Immunization.* The History of Vaccines. https://www.historyofvaccines.org/content/articles/future-immunization.

The Urgent Need For A National Plan To Contain The Coronavirus: Hearings before the Subcommittee on the Coronavirus Crisis, 116th Cong. (2020) (testimony of Anthony Fauci)

Thompson, D. (2020, May 6). *What's Behind South Korea's COVID-19 Exceptionalism?.* The Atlantic. https://www.theatlantic.com/ideas/archive/2020/05/whats-south-koreas-secret/611215/

Tian, J.-H., Patel, N., Haupt, R., Zhou, H., Weston, S., Hammond, H., Lague, J., Portnoff, A. D., Norton, J., Guebre-Xabier, M., Zhou, B., Jacobson, K., Maciejewski, S., Khatoon, R., Wisniewska, M., Moffitt, W., Kluepfel-Stahl, S., Ekechukwu, B., Papin, J., … Smith, G. (2020). SARS-CoV-2 spike glycoprotein vaccine candidate NVX-CoV2373 elicits immunogenicity in baboons and protection in mice. https://doi.org/10.1101/2020.06.29.178509

Tiberghien, P., Lamballerie, X. de, Morel, P., Gallian, P., Lacombe, K., & Yazdanpanah, Y. (n.d.). Collecting and evaluating convalescent plasma for COVID-19 treatment: Why and how? *Vox Sanguinis, n/a*(n/a). https://doi.org/10.1111/vox.12926

Tomita, K., Sakurai, F., Tachibana, M., & Mizuguchi, H. (2012). Correlation between adenovirus-neutralizing antibody titer and adenovirus vector-mediated transduction efficiency following intratumoral injection. *Anticancer Research, 32*(4), 1145–1152.

U.S. DEPARTMENT OF HEALTH AND HUMAN SERVICES, & NIH, N. I. of H., Understanding vaccines: what they are, how they work2–43 (2008). Bethesda, MD; U.S. Dept. of Health and Human Services, National Institutes of Health, National Institute of Allergy and Infectious Diseases.

U.S. Food & Drug Administration. (2020, June 30). *Coronavirus (COVID-19) Update: FDA Takes Action to Help Facilitate Timely Development of Safe, Effective COVID-19 Vaccines.* U.S. Food & Drug Administration. https://www.fda.gov/news-events/press-announcements/coronavirus-covid-19-update-fda-takes-action-help-facilitate-timely-development-safe-effective-covid

United Kingdom population mid-year estimate. (2020, June 24). Office for National Statistics. https://www.ons.gov.uk/peoplepopulationandcommunity/populationandmigration/populationestimates/timeseries/ukpop/pop

United Nations. (2020, April 17). *Ceasefire during COVID-19 pandemic essential, to safeguard 250 million children.* UN News. https://news.un.org/en/story/2020/04/1061962.

University of Arizona. (2000). *Antibody Structure.* The Biology Project. http://www.biology.arizona.edu/immunology/tutorials/antibody/structure.html.

Ura, T., Okuda, K., & Shimada, M. (2014). Developments in Viral Vector-Based Vaccines. *Vaccines, 2*(3), 624–641. https://doi.org/10.3390/vaccines2030624

Vaccines for children at school. (2015, August 28). Ontario.Ca. https://www.ontario.ca/page/vaccines-children-school

Valk, S. J., Piechotta, V., Chai, K. L., Doree, C., Monsef, I., Wood, E. M., Lamikanra, A., Kimber, C., McQuilten, Z., So-Osman, C., Estcourt, L. J., & Skoetz, N. (2020). Convalescent plasma or hyperimmune immunoglobulin for people with COVID-19: A rapid review. *Cochrane Database of Systematic Reviews, 5.* https://doi.org/10.1002/14651858.CD013600

Vartak, A., & Sucheck, S. (2016). Recent Advances in Subunit Vaccine Carriers. *Vaccines, 4*(2), 12. https://doi.org/10.3390/vaccines4020012

Wan, Y., Shang, J., Sun, S., Tai, W., Chen, J., Geng, Q., He, L., Chen, Y., Wu, J., Shi, Z., Zhou, Y., Du, L., Li, F. (2019). Molecular Mechanism for Antibody-Dependent Enhancement of Coronavirus Entry. *Journal of Virology, 94*(5). https://doi.org/10.1128/jvi.02015-19

Wang, J. M., Vardeny, O., & Zorek, J. A. (2016). High-dose influenza vaccine in older adults. *Journal of the American Pharmacists Association, 56*(1), 95–97. https://doi.org/10.1016/j.japh.2015.12.001

Wang, M., Jiang, S., & Wang, Y. (2016). Recent advances in the production of recombinant subunit vaccines in Pichia pastoris. *Bioengineered, 7*(3), 155–165. https://doi.org/10.1080/21655979.2016.1191707

Wang, N., Shi, X., Jiang, L., Zhang, S., Wang, D., Tong, P., Guo, D., Fu, L., Cui, Y., Liu, X., Arledge, K. C., Chen, Y.-H., Zhang, L., & Wang, X. (2013). Structure of MERS-CoV spike receptor-binding domain complexed with human receptor DPP4. *Cell Research, 23*(8), 986–993. https://doi.org/10.1038/cr.2013.92

Wang, Q., Zhang, Y., Wu, L., Niu, S., Song, C., Zhang, Z., Lu, G.,

Qiao, C., Hu, Y., Yuen, K.-Y., Wang, Q., Zhou, H., Yan, J., & Qi, J. (2020). Structural and Functional Basis of SARS-CoV-2 Entry by Using Human ACE2. *Cell*, *181*(4), 894-904.e9. https://doi.org/10.1016/j.cell.2020.03.045

Which COVID-19 Vaccines Are Being Developed with Aborted Babies? (2020, June 4). PRI. https://www.pop.org/which-covid-19-vaccines-are-being-developed-with-fetal-cell-lines-derived-from-aborted-babies/

Wiedermann, U., Garner-Spitzer, E., & Wagner, A. (2016). Primary vaccine failure to routine vaccines: Why and what to do? *Human Vaccines & Immunotherapeutics*, *12*(1), 239–243. https://doi.org/10.1080/21645515.2015.1093263

Woelfel, R., Corman, V. M., Guggemos, W., Seilmaier, M., Zange, S., Mueller, M. A., Niemeyer, D., Vollmar, P., Rother, C., Moelscher, M., Bliecker, T., Bruenink, S., Schneider, J., Elmann, R., Zwirglmaier, K., Drosten, C., Wendtner, C. (2020). Clinical presentation and virological assessment of hospitalized cases of coronavirus disease 2019 in a travel-associated transmission cluster. https://doi.org/10.1101/2020.03.05.20030502

World Health Organization. (2003, July 11). *Cumulative number of reported probable cases of SARS*. World Health Organization. https://www.who.int/csr/sars/country/2003_07_11/en/

World Health Organization. (2011, May 30). *Origin and development of health cooperation*. World Health Organization. https://www.who.int/global_health_histories/background/en/.

World Health Organization. (2012, April 13). *Health as a Bridge for Peace - HUMANITARIAN CEASE-FIRES PROJECT (HCFP)*. World Health Organization. https://www.who.int/hac/techguidance/hbp/cease_fires/en/.

World Health Organization. (2013, February 19). *Six common misconceptions about immunization*. World Health Organization. https://www.who.int/vaccine_safety/initiative/detection/immunization_misconceptions/en/index2.html.

World Health Organization. (2016, May 27). *Zika virus outbreak global response*. World Health Organization. https://www.who.int/emergencies/zika-virus/response/report/en/.

World Health Organization. (2017, December 5). *Smallpox vaccines*. World Health Organization. https://www.who.int/csr/disease/smallpox/vaccines/en/.

World Health Organization. (2020a, July 15). *New Zealand takes early and hard action to tackle COVID-19.* World Health Organization. https://www.who.int/westernpacific/news/feature-stories/detail/new-zealand-takes-early-and-hard-action-to-tackle-covid-19

World Health Organization. (2020b, June 26). *Key criteria for the ethical acceptability of COVID-19 human challenge studies.* World Health Organization. https://www.who.int/ethics/publications/key-criteria-ethical-acceptability-of-covid-19-human-challenge/en/.

World Health Organization. (n.d.). *The power of vaccines: Still not fully utilized.* World Health Organization. http://www.who.int/publications/10-year-review/vaccines/en/

World Health Organization. *Live Attenuated Vaccines (LAV). Vaccine Safety Basics.* World Health Organization. https://vaccine-safety-training.org/live-attenuated-vaccines.html.

Wu, K. J. (2020, July 21). *Some Vaccine Makers Say They Plan to Profit From Coronavirus Vaccine.* The New York Times. https://www.nytimes.com/2020/07/21/health/covid-19-vaccine-coronavirus-moderna-pfizer.html

Yang, F., Shi, S., Zhu, J., Shi, J., Dai, K., & Chen, X. (2020). Analysis of 92 deceased patients with COVID-19. *Journal of Medical Virology.* https://doi.org/10.1002/jmv.25891

Yang, H. (2020, June 6). *Press Releases-SINOVAC - Supply Vaccines to Eliminate Human Diseases.* SINOVAC. http://www.sinovac.com/?optionid=754.

Ye, F., Xu, S., Rong, Z., Xu, R., Liu, X., Deng, P., Liu, H., Xu, X. (2020). Delivery of infection from asymptomatic carriers of COVID-19 in a familial cluster. *International Journal of Infectious Diseases, 94,* 133–138. https://doi.org/10.1016/j.ijid.2020.03.042

Yuki, K., Fujiogi, M., & Koutsogiannaki, S. (2020). COVID-19 pathophysiology: A review. *Clinical Immunology, 215,* 108427. https://doi.org/10.1016/j.clim.2020.108427

Zhang, C., Maruggi, G., Shan, H., & Li, J. (2019, March 19). Advances in mRNA vaccines for infectious diseases. *Frontiers in Immunology, 10*(594). http://doi.org/10.3389/fimmu.2019.00594

Zhang, J.-M., & An, J. (2007). Cytokines, Inflammation and Pain. *International Anesthesiology Clinics, 45*(2), 27–37. https://doi.org/10.1097/AIA.0b013e318034194e

Zhu, F.-C., Li, Y.-H., Guan, X.-H., Hou, L.-H., Wang, W.-J., Li, J. X., Wu, S. P., Wang, B. S., Wand, Z., Wang, L., Jia, S. Y., Jiang, H. D., Wang, L., Jiang, T., Hu, H., Gou, J. B., Xu, S. B., Xu, J. J., Wang, X. W., … Chen, W. (2020). Safety, tolerability, and immunogenicity of a recombinant adenovirus type-5 vectored CO-VID-19 vaccine: a dose-escalation, open-label, non-randomised, first-in-human trial. *The Lancet*, *395*(10240), 1845–1854. https://doi.org/10.1016/s0140-6736(20)31208-3

Zucker, J. R., Rosen, J. B., Iwamoto, M., Arciuolo, R. J., Langdon-Embry, M., Vora, N. M., Rakeman, J. L., Isaac, B. M., Jean, A., Asfaw, M., Hawkins, S. C., Merrill, T. G., Kennelly, M. O., Maldin Morgenthau, B., Daskalakis, D. C., & Barbot, O. (2020). Consequences of Undervaccination—Measles Outbreak, New York City, 2018–2019. *New England Journal of Medicine*, *382*(11), 1009–1017. https://doi.org/10.1056/NEJMoa1912514

www.ingramcontent.com/pod-product-compliance
Lightning Source LLC
Chambersburg PA
CBHW030839270326
41928CB00007B/1128